The Ethics of Autism

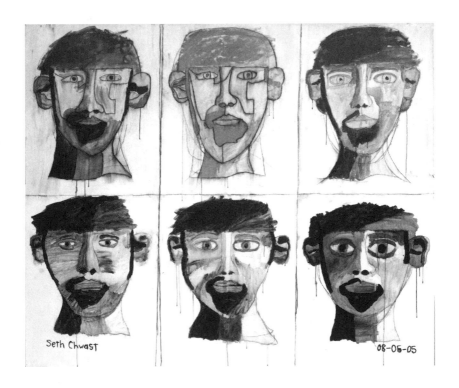

Seth Chwast

08-05-05

SETH CHWAST, *SIX SELF-PORTRAITS*

Bioethics and the Humanities

Eric M. Meslin and Richard B. Miller, editors

the ethics
of autism

Among Them, but Not of Them

Deborah R. Barnbaum

Indiana University Press
Bloomington & Indianapolis

All art courtesy of Fuchs and Kasperek, Inc.

This book is a publication of

Indiana University Press
601 North Morton Street
Bloomington, IN 47404-3797 USA

http://iupress.indiana.edu

Telephone orders	800-842-6796
Fax orders	812-855-7931
Orders by e-mail	iuporder@indiana.edu

The paper used in this publication meets the minimum requirements of American National Standard for Information Sciences—Permanence of Paper for Printed Library Materials, ANSI Z39.48-1984.

Manufactured in the United States of America

Library of Congress Cataloging-in-Publication Data

Barnbaum, Deborah R., date
  The ethics of autism : among them, but not of them / Deborah R. Barnbaum.
    p. ; cm. — (Bioethics and the humanities)
  Includes bibliographical references and index.
  ISBN 978-0-253-35213-2 (cloth : alk. paper) — ISBN 978-0-253-22013-4 (pbk. : alk. paper) 1. Autism—Philosophy. 2. Autism—Moral and ethical aspects. I. Title. II. Series.
  [DNLM: 1. Autistic Disorder—psychology. 2. Biomedical Research—ethics. 3. Mental Health Services—ethics. 4. Patient Care—ethics. 5. Philosophy, Medical. 6. Psychological Theory. WM 203.5 B256e 2008]
  RC553.A88B3657 2008
  616.85'882001—dc22
                                                             2008004040

2 3 4 5 13 12 11 10 09

For Michael

I stood
Among them, but not of them; in a shroud
Of thoughts which were not their thoughts.

LORD BYRON, *CHILDE HAROLD'S PILGRIMAGE*, CANTO II, STANZA 113

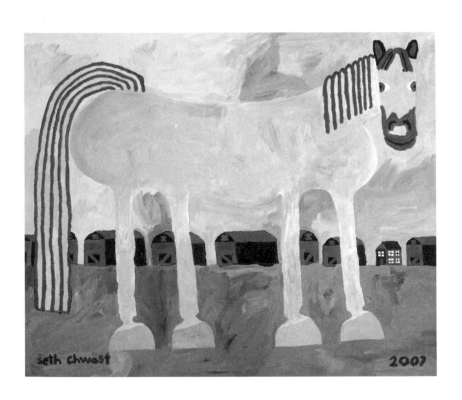

SETH CHWAST, *YELLOW-GREEN FANTASY HORSE*

Contents

Acknowledgments

My interest in philosophy and autism is long-standing. For that reason I have many people to thank for the transformation of that interest into this book. The editorial board and staff at Indiana University Press were enormously helpful. I owe thanks to Anne Clemmer for being available to answer every question. Robert A. Crouch, Miki Bird, and Marvin Keenan put in great time and attention at each editing phase. The book's design and incorporation of Seth Chwast's stunning images were accomplished beautifully by Jamison Cockerham. My greatest thanks at Indiana University Press are reserved for the editorial director, Robert J. Sloan.

Valuable insights of the students enrolled in my spring of 2005 graduate seminar on philosophy and autism were incorporated into the first three chapters of this book. Those students are Joseph Bocchicchio, Caemeron Crain, Alexander Cox, Brianna Miller, and David Schrapee.

Intellectual assistance from my colleagues in the Philosophy Department at Kent State University was substantial. Each of them was helpful, although a few deserve special mention. Deborah C. Smith's helpful suggestions contributed to a clearer presentation of material in the first chapter, in particular the material on philosophy of language. Linda Williams offered insights that allowed the discussion in the second chapter to take a more cogent turn. Susan Roxburgh, a colleague in the Sociology Department, offered suggestions that improved each "Voices of Autism" section. In addition to these contributions, support from and discussions with the remaining SB's—my good friends

Martha Cutter, Jeff Kriedler, Robert Trogdon, and Gina Zavota—were innumerable and invaluable. Julie Aultman, my colleague and friend at the Northeastern Ohio Universities College of Medicine, offered insight, as well as her personal library.

Kent State University granted me substantial time to complete this project, awarding me sabbatical leave in fall of 2005, as well as a Research and Creative Activity Award given by the Division of Research and Graduate Studies in spring 2006. I greatly appreciate Kent State University's dedication to faculty research.

My family, and in particular my father and my sister, have always been remarkably supportive, for which I am very grateful.

My husband, colleague, and closest friend, Gene Pendleton, deserves the most thanks for his indefatigable willingness to discuss autism, philosophy, and bioethics during the time I worked on this project. He read every word of this manuscript; his efforts improved my work in every aspect. His intellectual and emotional support means more than I can possibly articulate.

This book is dedicated to my brother, Michael, the hardest-working man with the keenest sense of justice that I know. This book would not have existed without him.

The Ethics of Autism

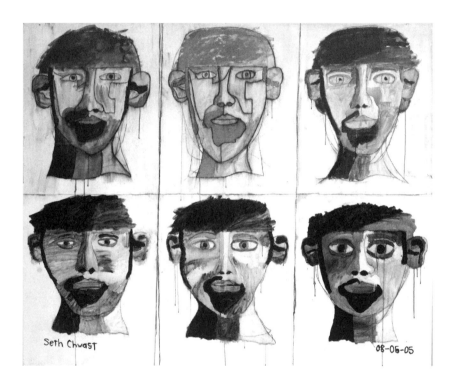

SETH CHWAST, *SIX SELF-PORTRAITS*

Introduction

Imagine if your understanding of other people was radically different from the way it is today. Picture a life where your understanding of the physical presence of other people is intact, but your sense of qualities such as beliefs, intentions, hopes, and speculations came fitfully, or perhaps only with great effort after a great deal of practice, or perhaps not at all. That life would be dramatically different from what most of us experience, since ascriptions of intentionality to others are so fundamental to our ways of thinking as well as our actions. Relationships with other persons are fundamental to who we are, how we come to understand ourselves, and even to what we believe constitutes a good life for ourselves. Who would you be if your experience of other people were significantly different than what you experience today?

Philosophers recognize that there is a sense in which none of us can know with certainty of the existence of other minds.[1] While we may not have direct evidence that other people have minds, we believe, and we have every reason to suspect, that other humans have intentions, such as beliefs, desires, wants, or fears. Most people behave as if other people had intentions, even though knowing with certainty that people do have intentions is a notoriously challenging philosophical problem. For years philosophers have been intrigued by the notion of persons who are unaware that other persons have minds. The existence of a mental solipsist—an individual who exists as the sole bearer of mind and mental states—was posited as the inevitable conclusion of epistemological theories unable to securely ground knowledge of the existence of other minds.

Imagine the person who does not ascribe intentionality to others in the way that most people do. How would such a person treat other people, and how would others treat him? What kind of life would that be for a person who does not recognize in a fundamental sense that other persons are out there?

Questions about the lives of persons who fail to have a rich understanding of others' intentionality serve as precursors to questions in normative theory about how we treat others, and how others treat us. Normative theory, in turn, acts as a precursor to applied questions, such as questions about the use of genetic technologies, or the use of humans in research. Before these questions in ethics can be answered, it makes sense first to understand the implications of a life of impoverished ascriptions of intentionality. There was a time when the notion of a person who did not recognize that other people had intentions was just an interesting thought experiment, a clever counterexample to philosophical theories. But psychologists have demonstrated that much more is at stake than fanciful objections to philosophical positions.

One explanation of the fundamental deficit facing persons with autism is the failure to attribute independent mental states to others. In other words, most persons with autism do not have a functioning "Theory of Mind." It is important to recognize that according to this view persons with autism are not merely *mistaken* about the content of the intentions that they ascribe to others. Because persons do not have direct access to others' intentions, it is not particularly novel that a person would be wrong about the intentions he ascribed to someone else. Even individuals who effortlessly ascribe intentions to persons are often wrong about the content of intentional states they ascribe to others ("But I thought you loved radishes!," "I did not bring the directions because I thought you knew how to get to the party!"). Rather, persons with autism are often challenged by ascriptions to others of *any* intentional states *at all*. The claim that persons with autism lack a theory of mind means that persons with autism are unable to employ certain types of intentional ascriptions, and in some cases are unable to recognize that other persons have a mental life separate from their own. Even those who believe that the fundamental deficit facing persons with autism is not the absence of a theory of mind, but rather a failure of executive function or central coherence, concede that these failures can result in the same difficulty with ascriptions of intentional states as the absence of a functioning theory of mind. Only after the full metaphysical ramifications of an autistic life are understood can we then grapple with the ethical implications of an autistic life.

According to Franz Brentano, intentionality is the defining criteria for something to be mental (Brentano 1973). In other words, mental states by their very nature are intentional. Intentionality encompasses not merely the mental phenomena of intentions, but also beliefs, desires, loves, hates, hopes, and fears. Intentionality is a complex and unique phenomenon, for many reasons. First, some intentional states, such as beliefs, have truth-values—what you believe can be true or false. The belief 'the ball is in the basket' may be true or false. Since intentional states are *about* things in a way that baskets or boxes are not, they are semantically evaluable. Second, while an agent can believe something to be true, it may be the case *that* the belief itself is false. Sally can believe that the ball is in the basket, but she may be mistaken, since the ball is actually in the box. Thus, a person who ascribes an intentional state to another person, S, is able to recognize that in some cases *it is true that S believes something that is false.* Third, intentional states including beliefs, desires, fears, or wants have causal powers: they can cause agents to perform actions. Sally looks for the ball in the basket in part because she *believes* that the ball is in the basket. Agents typically ascribe intentionality to other agents, taking what Daniel Dennett called the "intentional stance" toward others (Dennett 1987).

An individual who had difficulty in ascribing intentional states to others would have difficulty with all three of the above aspects of intentional states, with remarkable consequences. Consider, for example, beliefs. Given that intentional states are semantically evaluable, that it is possible for people to have both true and false beliefs, and that those (false) beliefs have causal powers, it is possible to assess a person's competence with at least some intentional ascriptions by evaluating his ability to understand the concept of a *false belief.* False-belief tests in which persons are asked to consider whether others hold false beliefs are widely used to evaluate the extent to which test subjects have a functioning theory of mind. Sally might look for the ball in the basket based on her false belief that the ball is in the basket, even though the ball is actually in the box. But an individual who lacks a functioning theory of mind and at the same time knows that the ball is actually in the box would be unable to predict Sally's actions based upon her false beliefs. Without a theory of mind the notion that Sally holds a false belief would escape him. A consequence of the causal efficacy of intentions is that persons who have difficulty ascribing intentionality to others would also find the behavior of others mysterious in many cases. Causal explanations of others' actions would not be available through conventional means. Combined, the three aspects of intentionality would render even straightforward explanations of behavior, such as "Sally looked in the basket because that's where she believed the ball to be (even though it is really in the box!)," problematic for someone who did not have a working theory of mind.

These three aspects of intentionality, and the implications for both philosophy of mind and philosophy of language of the fact that some lack a theory of mind, have piqued the curiosity of philosophers for over a decade. While autism raises questions in philosophy of mind and philosophy of language, comparatively few philosophers consider the implications of these unique deficits for ethics and for bioethics in particular. This book traces the philosophical questions raised by autism, from philosophy of mind and philosophy of language, through questions about moral personhood and what constitutes a well-lived human life, to questions about ethical theories practiced by persons with autism, and finally to the bioethical questions of the use of genetic technologies and the use of persons with autism as research subjects. The inquiry is driven by autism's uniqueness among disabilities. Some disabilities, such as paralysis or blindness, affect the ability to interact with the physical world, or require innovative strategies to interact with either physical objects or persons. Some conditions affect a person's longevity, or require a person to take medications, or deal with chronic pain. The significance of these disabilities, and their effects on the persons who have these disabilities, should not be understated. But autism is unique in that the absence of a functioning theory of mind carries with it the most profound implications for the ways in which persons with autism interact with others, or even come to understand themselves. In an anecdote that may ultimately be apocryphal, Helen Keller is quoted as saying that deafness is worse than blindness, because while blindness separates a person from objects, deafness separates a person from other people.[2] Although it is true that a deaf person can in some respects be cut off from a room full of hearing people, that deaf person nonetheless recognizes that there are persons from whom she is isolated. People who are deaf recognize that other people have intentional states.[3] Since autism results in a failure to recognize independent intentional states in others, the separation from other people that characterizes autism is more profound. The lack of a theory of mind among those with autism carries far-reaching philosophical implications.

Each of the following chapters begins with a portrait of an adult with autism, taken from that person's own writings. While each individual's autobiographical writing presents a richly faceted portrayal of autism, the portraits in this volume focus primarily on some of the philosophical themes in the respective chapters.

Chapter 1 begins by reviewing three prevailing theories of the primary deficit in autism. Just as applied ethics must be informed by normative theory, so too must applied and normative ethics be informed by empirical research. The first of these theories of autism is the *theory of mind* thesis, which holds that autism is characterized by the failure to recognize intentional states in others. The second thesis is the *weak central coherence* thesis, which holds that autism is best characterized by a failure to see coherent wholes. The weak central coherence thesis holds that persons with autism take a primarily detail-oriented approach, to the detriment of their ability to see coherent wholes. The third theory is the *weak executive function* thesis, which holds that autism is best described as a failure of planning and sorting, as well as the inability to switch from one task to another. All three of these theories are described, and evidence is offered both for and against each theory. While the theories are conceptually distinct, there is substantial phenomenological overlap among them. Most significantly, while the truth of the theory of mind thesis is not a foregone conclusion, the claim that persons with autism have tremendous difficulty ascribing intentionality to others is both empirically proven, and is consistent with the other two theories. The rest of the book takes facts about the failure to ascribe intentionality as its jumping-off point. Whichever explanation best accounts for autism, the fact that autism challenges a person's ability to make intentional ascriptions presents startling ethical implications.

Chapter 1 then proceeds with a philosophical examination of this failure to ascribe intentionality. Four significant questions in philosophy of mind and philosophy of language are considered. The first is this: does autism tell us anything about the theory theory versus simulation theory debate? Theory theory and simulation theory present alternative conceptions of the means by which agents explain others' actions. On the theory theory account, agents' actions are explained by ascribing beliefs and desires—theories, as it were—with the assumption that the agents act in keeping with those theories. On the simulation theory account, no "theories" are ascribed to the agents; instead, observers explain agents' actions by simulating what the observer would do in the position of the person whose behavior is being explained. That simulation is the basis for the explanation of others' actions. The strengths and weaknesses of theory theory and simulation theory are considered, as well as the failure of both as possible explanations given by autistic persons of others' actions. If the autistic person does not take the intentional stance toward others, theory theory is directly challenged. Simulation theory is faced with a less direct, but no less debilitating challenge. The nature of self-consciousness is the second philosophical question considered in chapter 1. Some philosophers believe that the failure to ascribe intentions to others may compromise our ability to ascribe intentions to ourselves. Might the failure of an autistic individual to take the intentional stance toward others affect his ability to take that stance toward himself? The ramifications of a lack of a theory of mind for self-consciousness are explored. Third, some meaning theories in philosophy of language are challenged by individuals who *are* competent language users, and yet are unable to take the intentional stance toward others. Both Gricean and Davidsonian meaning theories make use of agents' understanding of other agents' intentions, either directly or indirectly. There are persons with autism who are competent language users, yet who fail false-belief tasks designed to assess their theory of mind. Autism's challenges to these theories of meaning are examined. Finally, chapter 1 concludes with an examination of the modularity of mind thesis. Some philosophers have speculated that the mind is separated into modules. Does autism tell us anything about whether a theory of mind module exists?

These issues in philosophy of mind and philosophy of language secure a foundation from which to ask ethical questions about autism. Given the conclusions in philosophy of mind and language, the autistic person might appear to be on tenuous moral ground. Some claim that entering into interpersonal relationships, those that are only available to persons with a theory of mind, is essential to membership in the moral community, thereby calling into question the moral status of autistic individuals. Chapter 2 addresses the following question: what is the moral standing of a person with autism? Many philosophers have speculated on questions about moral status and personhood. Different approaches to moral personhood, and the qualities of a well-lived human life, are considered. An exhaustive examination of these questions would be prohibitively long, but several contemporary discussions, from a variety of philosophical perspectives, are presented.

The first of these is Mary Ann Warren's discussion of membership in the moral community. Warren presents several criteria for membership in the moral community, some of which pose a difficulty for persons with autism. Second, Martha Nussbaum's discussion of human capabilities is examined. Nussbaum has considered the implications of her view for persons with disabilities. However, in light of the philosophical challenges of autism, Nussbaum's position deserves a closer look. Third, the theories of human well-being articulated by Derek Parfit, Thomas Scanlon, and Robert M. Veatch are examined. Each of these philosophers brings a different nuance to the debate. Their discussions are notable for the role played by objective goods, and for the role of relationships in particular to a good human life. Next, Peter Hobson's view on the human form of social life, and its implications for persons with autism, are examined. Hobson is the first of the philosophers in chapter 2 who directly addresses questions about persons with autism in light of their theory of mind difficulties. Piers Benn is another philosopher who addresses these questions directly and who presents the most controversial view entertained in the chapter: persons with autism are not members of the moral community. In light of the extreme nature of his view, his argument is examined in detail. While Benn's argument appears to be the logical extension of some of the positions advocated earlier, chapter 2 concludes by rejecting Benn's position. When others are excluded from the moral community, everyone suffers. It is actually *non-autistic persons* who are on tenuous moral ground when they attempt to exclude persons with autism from the moral community. Non-autistic persons exclude autistic persons from the moral community at their own peril.

Chapter 3 moves from questions about the value of autistic lives to a question about normative ethics: given the theory of mind deficits faced by the autistic individual, which moral theory can accommodate both autistic and non-autistic persons alike? Many moral theories are rejected because they rely too heavily on an agent's sense of empathy or community, both of which may be compromised for individuals with autism. For example, Jeannette Kennett speculates that a Humean moral theory relies too much on a sense of empathy to be useful to the autistic agent. Hume's moral theory is the first that is dismissed for its inability to bridge the gap between autistic and non-autistic agents. One of the vexing problems for utilitarianism—locating a motive to compel agents to act according to utilitarianism—is only further complicated by autistic agency. Kennett believes that while a Humean theory cannot work for the autistic agent, a Kantian theory may be more workable. Kennett's conclusions may be too hasty, however, since Kantian moral theory has its own stumbling blocks for autistic agents. Other moral theories, such as moral particularism, as well as an ethic of *prima facie* duties, are equally challenging. The inapplicability of an ethic of *prima facie* duties for autistic agents is especially troubling because one of the most prominent bioethical theories in use today, Tom Beauchamp and James F. Childress's theory, is an example of an ethic of *prima facie* duties.

If no shared moral theory among autistic and non-autistic agents can be agreed upon, then answers to applied questions will similarly elude mutual agreement. The moral divide between autistic and non-autistic agents is illustrated at the end of chapter 3 with a brief consideration of one applied ethical question: if a "cure" emerges for adults with autism, who should decide whether to administer it? Chapter 3 shows that many of the most well-established moral theories do not bridge the gap between the autistic and non-autistic populations, making the answers to this and other applied questions all the more confounding.

The administration of a possible "cure" to adults with autism only begins to scratch the surface of applied ethical questions that emerge when considering autism. Chapter 4 begins with a detailed discussion of the bioethical questions posed by autism. One debate concerns the use of genetic technologies and autism. At present, genetic tests are unable to determine whether an individual will be born with autism, although there is strong evidence for a genetic component in many cases. When genetic markers for autism are located, significant ethical dilemmas will also come to light. Should eventual genetic technologies be used to prevent the birth of future children with autism, or is such a use of genetic technologies morally impermissible? One argument examined is an argument from parental autonomy, which states that unlimited parental autonomy permits any decision about future children. This argument is presented, evaluated, and rejected. A second argument against the use of genetic technologies to prevent the birth of future persons with autism proceeds from assumptions about the social construction of disability. Based on claims in chapter 2, this argument is also rejected. A related argument examines the parallel between communities of persons with a disability, such as the Deaf community, and the community of persons with autism. However, in light of dissimilarities between these two communities, this argument is also rejected. The permissibility of using genetic technologies to prevent future persons from being born with autism is established by invoking and defending Joel Feinberg's right to an open future argument against its critics.

The use of genetic markers to identify who will or will not have autism may be remote, but a second option exists today which can allow at-risk families to lower their chances of having a child with autism. Given the four-to-one ratio of males to females among persons with autism, one course of action available to high-risk families is to use sex selection, that is, choosing to have a female child who is therefore less likely to have autism. Many bioethicists argue that sex selection is morally impermissible, but perhaps autism changes the ethical landscape with respect to sex selection. Should parents be permitted to use sex selection to prevent the birth of future autistic children? Arguments for and against this practice are considered. While there are significant reasons to disallow widespread sex selection, autism appears to be an ethical exception. The right to an open future argument is adopted to show that there are no good choices in these circumstances, but that the least bad option for at-risk families is to use sex selection in order to do what they can to help promote the best life for future persons.

Chapter 5 considers another question linking autism and bioethics: can we use persons with autism as biomedical research subjects? Behavioral and psychological research typically does not carry the risks of harms that biomedical research does, but it also does not hold out possible benefit of a cure, as does some biomedical research. But the status of this "benefit" may complicate the ethical terrain when it comes to research into autism. One question is whether biomedical research on human beings should be permitted at all. The utilitarian and ethic of *prima facie* duties arguments for, as well as the Kantian argument against, the use of humans in research are considered. Given the discussion in chapter 3, it would appear that none of these arguments is convincing with respect to autistic persons. Competency to consent to research is then examined. Traditional conceptions of competency, such as that proposed by Allen Buchanan and Dan W. Brock, are problematic for persons with autism. More flexible accounts, though, such as the goodness-of-fit ethic proposed by Celia B. Fisher, are also challenged by the autistic research subject. Competency to offer informed consent to participate in research may be beyond some autistic persons. If biomedical research is performed on persons with autism, proxy decision making may be the only option left.

Proxy consent by surrogates is typically justified on the basis of two standards: the substituted judgment standard or the best interest standard. The substituted judgment standard is shown to be inapplicable for the incompetent person with autism; thus, the best interest standard is considered in detail. Here, the ethical complications of biomedical research that may directly benefit persons with autism are fully revealed. The ethical questions surrounding a "cure" for autism, first considered in chapter 3, are revisited. An argument is considered about biomedical research on adults with autism that may hold out the direct benefit of a "cure." The argument brings together several of the most vexing questions in bioethics—therapeutic versus non-therapeutic research, greater-than-minimal-risk research on non-autonomous research subjects, research that holds out the prospect of merely aspirational rather than direct benefits. Given points made earlier, it would appear that such research is not ethically permissible on the basis of a best interest standard of proxy consent. The unique deficits faced by persons with autism make it the case that it is not necessarily beneficial to adults with autism to be cured. Adults with autism should be permitted to live out their lives without the threat of being cured, even in the course of research studies.

This starling position leads to the last point in the book—a call for autistic integrity. Adults with autism should be respected as persons who are leading a life that is different—in some ways incomprehensibly different—from the life led by those who are not autistic. But to try to change the autistic adult into someone who is not autistic is to fail to respect him as a person in his own right. A call for autistic integrity requires the non-autistic population to recognize that adults with autism have distinct personalities, preferences, and pleasures just as any non-autistic adult does; to try to "cure" them of autism is to fundamentally change who they are in a way that denies them the respect they deserve.

Autistic and non-autistic people are equally among—but not of—each other. Their ways of thinking are equally opaque to one another. How this is so, and what this means for questions in bioethics is the subject of this book.

Voices of Autism

Jim Sinclair *wrote an autobiographical essay, "Bridging the Gaps: An Inside-Out View of Autism (Or, Do You Know What I Don't Know?)," at the age of twenty-seven. Sinclair did not use speech to communicate until he was twelve years old, and did not have a vocabulary to articulate his own feelings until he was twenty-five. He attributes this delay to the fact that no one explained to him what the words for subjective experiences actually meant until he was much older. He recounts the painstaking way in which he needed to learn and relearn words and their meanings, relearning to read numerous times, and not always having the certainty that the words he would hope to use were available to him (Sinclair 1992, 298).*

Sinclair's observations of an autistic life run the gamut from reflections on self-consciousness to relationships with others. Sinclair's assessment is that autism means that his "input-output equipment may work in nonstandard ways" (Sinclair 1992, 295), including the ability to extract meaning out of language. For this reason, Sinclair says that persons with autism might have to learn what other people seem to know without learning, such as evidencing feelings by not just using words, but by having those feelings reflected in facial expressions. While spoken language and the complex language of relationships present difficulties, Sinclair holds that he is "never out of touch with my core" (Sinclair 1992, 298). His own mental states may be difficult to articulate to others, but his reflections on his own conscious states are uncompromised.

Sinclair's observations about the role of relationships in his life are richly nuanced. On one hand, he observes that there are times when he is comfortable going days or weeks without having contact with other people.

Even those long stretches of being alone do not result in loneliness. Sinclair admits that there are some aspects of human relationships that are baffling to him, requiring a "separate translation code for every person I meet" (Sinclair 1992, 300), because social cues can escape him. On the other hand, indifference to relationships frees him to form attachments only with those people whose company he truly enjoys. This freedom, combined with the fact that he needs a separate translation code for each person, distinguishes his connections with those people with whom he chooses to associate. The intensity of the attachment may be rich, and not merely a pale imitation of non-autistic connections. Despite this intensity, Sinclair observes that his connections with other people can be transient. "I don't stick," he says (Sinclair 1992, 301).

Sinclair concludes his essay with this observation: "My personhood is intact. My selfhood is undamaged. I find great value and meaning in my life, and I have no wish to be cured of being myself" (Sinclair, p. 302).

1

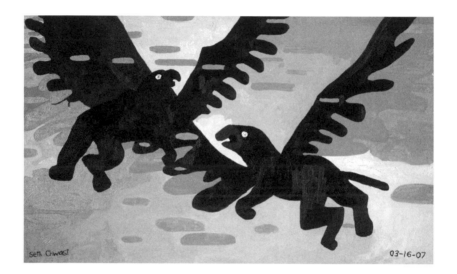

SETH CHWAST, 2 BLACK GRIFFINS ON VALENTINE'S DAY SKY

A Philosophical Introduction to Autism

This chapter lays the groundwork for a subsequent discussion of ethics and autism. In order to understand the ethical implications of this complex disorder, an understanding of autism is essential. Three predominant theories of autism are considered: the theory of mind thesis, the weak central coherence thesis, and the weak executive function thesis. Evidence for each of these theories is presented. Where it is possible, common ground among these competing accounts is noted.

Second, a discussion is presented of four problems that emerge when considering autism in philosophy of mind, and philosophy of language. The unique character of autism plays a significant role with respect to the theory theory versus simulation theory debate, the nature of self-consciousness, meaning theory in philosophy of language, and the notion of modularity of mind. In some cases, autism poses a challenge to long-held philosophical positions. In other cases, autism presents itself as empirical support to bolster the plausibility of one theory over another. In the case of the theory theory and simulation theory debate, autism arises as a challenge to both prevailing theories. Neither theory theory nor simulation theory are available to autistic agents to explain the behavior of others, but evidence from autism is cited to support one of these theories over the other. In the case of theories of self-consciousness, autism poses a challenge to the belief that while we do not have direct access to others' consciousness, we at least have direct access to our own. Autism may present a novel account of self-consciousness. With respect to philosophy of language, speakers with autism pose a counterexample both to theories that postulate that meaning depends on speakers' and listeners' intentions, as well as theories that claim meaning is tied to interpretation among speakers and listeners. Finally, proponents of the mental module theory of the mind will look to the possibility of a theory of mind module as evidence for their theory, although the evidence from autism is mixed.

One more interesting philosophical question can be raised: what implications follow for each of these four areas in the philosophy of mind and philosophy of language in ethical theory and for bioethics? The implications may not be immediately obvious, but in time their significance will become clear. The discussion in chapter 2 about personhood and well-lived human lives makes significant use of claims about the value of consciousness and self-consciousness. Arguments about the inapplicability of David Hume's moral theory for autistic agents in chapter 3 turn on the use of simulation theory. Arguments about an ethic of *prima facie* duties in chapter 3 have much in common with claims about autistic speakers' use of pragmatics in language. The Deaf community argument in chapter 4 about the use of genetic technologies makes use of the concept of "community," yet the shared experiences and interests of members of a given community may turn, at least in part, on shared understandings of actions, activities, and communication. A method of explanation of others' behaviors, such as theory theory or simulation theory, or shared meaning when using language, should be available to members of a community. If an agent does not understand others well enough to explain their actions, or cannot engage in shared communication, in what sense can that agent share something as significant as "community" with others? These are only a few examples of foundational questions in philosophy of mind, or philosophy of language, informing ethical considerations. Understanding the full range of autism's ethical complexities first necessitates understanding the philosophical implications in philosophy of mind and philosophy of language. And understanding the *philosophical* complexities of autism first necessitates understanding the nature of autism itself.

The Theory of Mind Thesis of Autism, and Competing Theories

Three accounts of autism are of particular interest to philosophers.[1] The first of these accounts is the theory of mind thesis. The second is the weak central coherence thesis. The third is the weak executive function thesis. Many of the conclusions in this book follow from interesting consequences of the theory of mind thesis, although the others bear mention for two reasons. First, if there are significant theories in addition to the theory of mind thesis, they should be examined. Blithely assuming that there is only one significant theory—coincidentally, the theory that promotes the most interesting bioethical consequences—is not intellectually honest. Second, some believe that the theory of mind thesis is not incompatible with competing accounts. There is speculation that the theory of mind thesis must complement other accounts, as no one theory provides a complete explanation of all characteristics of autism. A stronger thesis holds that theory of mind deficits are a *result* of weak central coherence or weak executive function. Thus, competing accounts of autism may be compatible, or even support, many of the most interesting ethical conclusions.

All three of the theories attempt to explain the core deficits faced by persons with autism. According to the fourth edition of the American Psychiatric Association's *Diagnostic and Statistical Manual of Mental Disorders* (DSM-IV), psychiatry's principal diagnostic manual, autism is characterized by twelve diagnostic criteria which are divided into three major areas. A diagnosis of autism requires at least two signs from A, one sign each from B and C, and at least six signs overall (American Psychiatric Association 1994, 70–71):

A. Qualitative impairments in reciprocal social interaction as manifested by at least two of the following:
   i. impairment in multiple non-verbal behaviors such as eye-to-eye gaze and facial expression
   ii. failure to develop peer relationships appropriate to developmental level

          iii. lack of spontaneous seeking to share interests or enjoyments with others
          iv. lack of social or emotional reciprocity

  B. Qualitative impairments in communication
          i. delay, or lack or, development of spoken language
          ii. impairment in the ability to initiate or sustain conversation despite adequate speech
          iii. stereotyped and repetitive, or idiosyncratic, use of language
          iv. lack of varied spontaneous pretend play or social imitative play appropriate to developmental level

  C. Restricted, repetitive, and stereotyped patterns of behavior, interests, or activities
          i. preoccupation with one or more patterns of interest, with abnormal intensity or focus
          ii. compulsive adherence to nonfunctional routines or rituals
          iii. stereotyped or repetitive motor mannerisms
          iv. persistent preoccupation with parts of objects

In addition to the above symptoms, approximately 10 percent (Frith 2003) of persons with autism have what Leo Kanner referred to as "islets of ability"—special talents and abilities in areas as diverse as painting, music, or mathematics (Kanner 1943).

Asperger's syndrome, a condition closely related to autism, may be diagnosed when children show no delays in language acquisition or other cognitive development, although the social impairments and obsessions are still in evidence (Frith 2003). There is some dispute as to whether Asperger's and autism are distinct, or whether "both are variants of the same underlying developmental disorder" (Frith 2003, 11). While Asperger's syndrome has its own DSM criteria distinct from autism, Asperger's is believed to be "on the same 'spectrum' of neurologically-based social dysfunction as autism" (Siegel 1996, 113) and is often recognized as being similar to high-functioning autism. Three significant theories have emerged to explain what could account for the above combination of symptoms.

The Theory of Mind Thesis

One hypothesis is that the core deficits found in autism can be explained by the fact that persons with autism are not able to recognize that other persons have minds. To recognize that another person has a mind is to recognize that person as someone who has a mental life independent of your own, with beliefs, preferences, desires, and the whole range of intentional attitudes. There are two accounts of the failure of theory of mind. One account is that persons who lack a functioning theory of mind have difficulty ascribing intentional states to others at all. Thus, they are unable to take the intentional stance toward others. On another account, the failure of theory of mind could result in a mistaken attribution of the *autistic person's* intentional states to *all other* intentional agents. The state of affairs that would result would be akin to a "unified consciousness" view on the part of persons with autism—the mistaken belief that everyone shares the same intentional states as he does.[2]

Most discussions of the failure of theory of mind and autism embrace the first view, that people with autism are unable to take the intentional stance toward others. Persons with autism who fail to have a functioning theory of mind are therefore unable to make intentional ascriptions, or in some cases are hamstrung by making consistently inapt intentional ascriptions. There is a conceptual distinction between the failure to make intentional ascriptions at all, and the failure to recognize others as having intentions distinct from one's own (the unified consciousness view), but similar consequences may emerge in both cases: a lack of empathy, a failure to enter into relationships that embrace other persons *qua* persons, and the inability to enter into reciprocal relationships. Kanner's 1943 descriptions of "autistic aloneness" are apt and anticipate the theory of mind thesis: persons with autism are alone in that they fail to recognize that other persons, in a mental sense, exist. Simon Baron-Cohen calls these abnormalities in recognizing other minds "a core and possibly universal abnormality" of autistic spectrum disorders (Baron-Cohen 2000b, 3). The theory of mind thesis is compatible with other theories that present a physiological explanation for the deficits in autism. For example, recent attention has been paid to the "mirror neuron" theory, which postulates that autistic deficits are the result of misfires in neurons that are responsible for empathetic emotional responses (Ramachandran and Oberman 2006). These mirror neurons facilitate not only empathetic responses, but also the understanding of intentional states.

Uta Frith and Francesca Happé observe that "the litmus test for [theory of mind] has been the ability to attribute *false beliefs* to others" (Frith and Happé 1999, 3).[3] Several versions of false-belief tasks exist. One, the "Sally-Anne test," asks children to consider the following scenario. Sally and Anne, often represented by puppets, play with a marble, which they place in a basket. Sally then leaves the room, and Anne moves the marble from the basket into a box. After observing this, the test subject is asked "Where will Sally look for her marble?" or, in some cases, "Where will Sally think the marble is?" (Baron-Cohen 1995, 71). Children with an intact theory of mind will recognize that Sally will look for the marble where she last thought it was: in the basket. Sally has a false belief about where the marble is, even though the test subject has a true belief about the marble's location. Passing the false-belief task requires that the subject recognize that while he has a true belief, someone in Sally's position would nonetheless have a false belief. Children who fail to have a theory of mind don't recognize this, and instead answer that Sally will look for the marble where it in fact is—in the box. A second test of theory of mind is known as the "Smarties test." A child is shown a tube of Smarties candy and is asked what is in the tube. The child, recognizing the exterior of the tube, answers that the tube contains candy. When the tube is opened, it is revealed that the tube disappointingly contains only pencils. When typically developing children are asked what they initially thought was in the tube, and what someone outside the room might believe to be in the tube, the children answer correctly. With a functioning theory of mind, a child is able to recognize that a person outside the room, and not privy to the revealed contents of the tube, will answer as she initially did—the other person will have the false belief that the tube contains candy. Children with autism answer "pencils" to both of these questions. The incorrect answer demonstrates both an inability to reflect on their previous false beliefs, as well as an inability to correctly attribute false beliefs to others (Baron-Cohen 1995). Both of these tests are known as *first-order* false-belief tests, as they require the subject to make an inference about another person's belief states. *Second-order* false-belief tests require the subject to consider beliefs about beliefs: where does Anne think that Sally will look for the marble?

Typically developing children with an intact theory of mind are able to pass these false-belief tests with a great deal of accuracy by the age of three or four (Wimmer and Perner 1983). Children with Down syndrome are also able to pass these tests. But children with autism have a fairly significant failure rate on these false-belief tests (Baron-Cohen, 1995), including children with autism who have a higher "mental age" than the typically developing children or those with Down syndrome. The Sally-Anne test and the Smarties test examine the ability that subjects have to recognize first-order false beliefs—the fact that someone holds a false belief. Even those subjects with autism who are able to recognize first-order false beliefs—between 20 and 35 percent of children with autism are able to do so—have tremendous difficulty with second-order beliefs. Most teenagers with autism cannot correctly answer questions about second-order false beliefs, such as "Where does Anne think that Sally thinks the marble is?" (Baron-Cohen 1995).

The evidence from these false-belief tests has been cited as support for the claim that persons with autism have difficulty recognizing that other persons have mental lives, separate from their own. The ability to understand and anticipate other people's propositional attitudes is occasionally referred to as "mindreading," not in the sense of the paranormal, or extra-sensory perception, but rather in the sense that each typically developing individual is aware that others have a mental life, and is usually able to grasp what others might be thinking, given the right clues. This failure to mindread is believed to be one of the defining characteristics of autism:

> Mindreading deficits in autism spectrum conditions appear to be early occurring (from at least the end of the first year of life, if one includes joint attention deficits) and universal (if one tests for these either at the right point in development, or in the case of high-functioning, older subjects by using sensitive, age-appropriate tests). (Baron-Cohen 2000b, 16)

While the ability to mindread should not be seen as a diagnostic tool, the failure of theory of mind in autism is well-documented and is believed to be an accurate description of the underlying difficulty confronting persons with autism.

Kathrin Glüer and Peter Pagin observe that an essential step in folk psychological explanations is that an agent is able to ascribe beliefs to oneself and others; to do this, one must recognize that a belief can be *false,* even when held by oneself or by others: "To understand the difference between *being* true and being *believed* to be true, one must understand that a belief can be false, and this understanding is manifested by means of the ability to ascribe beliefs one takes to be false" (Glüer and Pagin 2003, 27).

If a person lacked a theory of mind, this could explain symptoms of autism such as social abnormalities as well as difficulties in language. Persons who lack a theory of mind would have difficulties with the notion that "seeing leads to knowing"—the fact that Sally was not in the room when the marble went into the box means that she does not know where the marble is. Without this understanding, persons with autism would have difficulty in communication, as they would have difficulty detecting what a hearer already knows, or what that hearer does not yet know (Baron-Cohen 2000b). Jill de Villiers (2000) claims that language ability is essential for an agent to ascribe false beliefs to others. Language is necessary for the concepts required to understand a false belief, such as "belief" or "think," and yet there is evidence on both sides as to which of the two—language competency or an understanding of false beliefs—is causally prior. Jay L. Garfield, Candida Peterson, and Tricia Perry (2001) hold that language competency and social competency are jointly sufficient and both causally necessary for theory of mind deficits. They cite evidence of deaf children raised by parents who are competent sign language users: those children demonstrate relative capacity with theory of mind concepts, as contrasted with the difficulty deaf children who are raised by hearing (that is, non-fluent signing) parents have with theory of mind concepts. The complexity of the relationship between language and theory of mind demonstrates that "the developmental relationship between language and theory of mind is not just one-way" (de Villiers 2000, 116). In her own research with children who are autistic and children who are deaf, de Villiers concludes that language is necessary for false-belief reasoning, and that this accounts for those deaf children who are lagging behind in communicative ability and performing poorly on false-belief tasks. However, de Villiers observes that children who only have a language delay do not also demonstrate the other deficits associated with a lack of theory of mind.

In addition to these aspects of theory of mind deficits, in which other persons would present a bit of a mystery, objects might be far less mysterious, and in fact, might hold a strange fascination. It has been suggested that the deficits in folk psychology that accompany the inability to read other people's minds could come in tandem with increased abilities in "folk physics" (Baron-Cohen 2000a). If the autistic individual finds people a mystery, he may direct his energies and attentions to objects, becoming an expert in non-intentional realms such as bus routes, astronomy, or antique watches. The "false-photo task," a counterpart to the false-belief task, demonstrates that many autistic people have superior abilities in these areas. In the false-photo task, a subject is first shown how a Polaroid camera works. A picture is then taken of a room in which a doll is sitting on a chair. After the picture is taken, the doll is moved. When asked "Where will the doll be in the picture?" children with autism answer the question with greater accuracy than do typically developing children. False beliefs are confounding to people with autism, but false photos present little problem. In the false-belief tasks, intentionality marks the difference between the correct and incorrect answer, but in false-photo tasks, none of the confounding elements inherent in intentionality is involved.

A further elaboration on the theory of mind thesis is the systematizing/empathizing account (Baron-Cohen 2003). According to this account, the typical male brain is more attuned to "systematizing" tasks, such as creating and modifying taxonomies. The typical female brain is more attuned to "empathizing" tasks, such as learning what others are thinking or feeling by reading the language of facial expressions, and in particular, the language of the eyes as well as the ability to respond "spontaneously in an emotionally appropriate way" (Lawson 2003,

191). These abilities stand in contrast with one another, with strengths in one appearing alongside deficits in the other (Happé 2000, 214). Autism, on this account, is understood as an extreme version of the male brain—autism renders someone adept at systematizing tasks, building with blocks, or pouring over bus schedules. The inability to empathize would result in unsociability, an autistic aloneness. The fact that autism is an example of an "extreme male brain" might also account for the overwhelming number of persons with autism being male: four in five persons with autism are male, and Asperger's affects males at ten times the rate as it does females (Siegel 1996, 12). Some measures place the ratio of males to females with Asperger's at fifteen to one (Frith 2003, 65). This account is not inconsistent with the theory of mind thesis, however. What it may mean to have a brain that systematizes well, but that does not empathize well, is that one is particularly adept at folk physics, but not adept at folk psychology. A person with an extreme male brain may be so poor at folk psychology that he is unable to forge the understanding that other persons have mental lives independent from his own. Baron-Cohen observes that interpersonal relationships are possible with higher-functioning persons with autism, but only on their own terms (Baron-Cohen 2003, 140). An appreciation of others' mental lives, desires, and preferences does not typically enter into the equation.

In summary, the theory of mind theory of autism seeks to explain the diagnostic criteria of autism by postulating that persons with autism fail to recognize the mental lives of others.[4] Such a failure would explain difficulties in social interaction and impairments in communication, as both of these are strongly tied to an understanding of other people. While the theory of mind theory may be on shakier ground explaining the restricted and repetitive patterns of behavior associated with autism, both the inclination of folk physics over folk psychology, and the systematizing versus empathizing brain theories go considerable distance toward accounting for these traits.

The Weak Central Coherence Thesis

Central coherence is the ability to see not merely parts, but wholes—the ability to draw together details so as to recognize the meaning of the entire picture. Persons with weak central coherence fail to see the whole, and instead will focus on details, even if those details are irrelevant to the significance of the whole. The ability to determine the meanings or pronunciations of homographs in context ("Her dress had a big tear in it" versus "Her eye had a big tear in it") is accounted for by central coherence. Proponents of the weak central coherence theory of autism "find that it is possible to explain the pattern of abilities in autism by a relatively simple and strong hypothesis: a tendency to weak central coherence" (Frith 2003, 161). It is also possible that weak central coherence would account for a local bias in the processing of information (Happé and Frith 2006). Some theorists have speculated that the failure on the Sally-Anne task is a result of weak central coherence. The detail that the marble is now in the box overwhelms an autistic child's mind, and the larger picture—that Sally left the room; that she left thinking the marble was one place whereas now it is somewhere else—is overwhelmed by the detail that *the marble is in fact in the basket*. This hypothesis is consistent with the one forwarded by Allan W. Snyder, that autism is understood as an absence of mental paradigms. Without mental paradigms—or "mindsets," as Snyder calls them—the world would be one of continual surprises, one in which "everything would have to be examined anew by treating each detail with equal importance" (Snyder 1998, 3).

Weak central coherence may explain certain obsessions held by persons with autism, as these obsessions are often detail-oriented. Weak central coherence may also account for strengths persons with autism show in finding embedded figures or creating designs out of segmented blocks (Frith 2003, 152–156). One of the advantages of a weak central coherence account is that it explains factors associated with autism that are not associated with mindreading (Happé 2000). Some philosophers have examined the weak central coherence thesis as an explanation of why children with autism succeed at the false-photo task, yet fail the false-belief task. Claire O'Loughlin and Paul

Thagard (2000) stake out the position that weak central coherence can be understood as a failure of "constraint satisfaction"—the ability to maximally resolve coherence and incoherence relations among concepts and propositions—and develop a model which ties failures on both false-belief tasks and failures on homographic tasks to these failures of constraint satisfaction. Deepthi Kamawar, Jay L. Garfield, and Jill de Villiers (2002) dispute O'Loughlin and Thagard's model and the weak central coherence thesis by arguing that this model proves too much, as it would predict that persons with autism would fail both false-belief tasks as well as false-photo tasks. The tasks, they argue, are isomorphic: both involve a scene which is changed in such a way that the change is not represented in the present visualization, and yet the participant must determine if the change is reflected in the original scene or only in the new scene (Kamawar et al. 2002, 269). Thagard and O'Loughlin's response (2002) is that the false-photo task and false-belief task are not isomorphic, and thus the success on false-photo tasks does not provide a counterexample to the weak central coherence theory of autism.

In summary, the weak central coherence thesis endeavors to explain each of the three characteristics of autism. Impairments in social interaction, deficits in communication, and repetitive behaviors might all be attributed to attention to detail to the detriment of the whole. Those who believe that the weak central coherence thesis and the theory of mind theory offer an incomplete picture of autism have a third theory available.

The Weak Executive Function Thesis

A third explanation of autism is that persons with autism have weak executive function. Executive function is what allows for planning and organization (Perner and Lang 2000), as well as "for keeping several tasks going at the same time and switching between them. They are vital for high-level decisions to resolve conflicting responses, for overriding automatic behavior, and for inhibiting inappropriate impulsive actions" (Frith 2003, 177–178). Weak executive function may account for repeated, stereotyped behavior on the part of some people with autism. It is possible that the failure on the Sally-Anne task may be accounted for by failing to switch from the recognition that the marble *actually is in the box* to the recognition that Sally would *think that the marble is still in the basket.* Shaun Nichols and Stephen Stich take experiments in which autistic children are not able to maintain a clear appearance/reality distinction as evidence that "Perhaps autistic children have difficulty updating their beliefs on the basis of new information; perhaps they perseverate on first impressions . . ." (Nichols and Stich 2003, 179). For example, there are experiments in which autistic children are shown a sponge that is made to look like a granite rock—the initial appearance indicates that the object is a rock, but the reality is that the object is a sponge. The children are ultimately shown that the object is in fact a sponge. However, even after being shown that the sponge is a sponge that merely looks like a rock, children with autism will tell questioners that the object is a rock, and not a sponge. Thus, the first impression stays with the children, even in the face of additional evidence. These experiments may lend support for a weak executive function theory of autism, as they demonstrate an inability to switch ideas based on new evidence. Individuals who are unable to pass false-belief tasks may know what it is to ascribe a false belief to others, but poor executive function makes it impossible for them to suppress their own true belief (Glüer and Pagin 2003). Thus the weak executive function hypothesis has much in common with the unified consciousness version of the theory of mind hypothesis.

Baron-Cohen, a proponent of the theory of mind thesis, observes that the weak executive function account is at pains to explain why typically developing two-year-olds can move easily in and out of pretend play, even though children of that same age find other executive function switching tasks so difficult (Baron-Cohen 2000b). It is unclear, also, how weak executive function might account for both failures in false-belief tests, and yet success in false-photo tests. A weak executive function thesis, however, does offer some explanation to account for many stereotyped behaviors such as rocking or hand flapping, as well as social and linguistic difficulties.

One of the reasons that there are competing accounts is that no one theory appears to explain all aspects of autism—"autism has defied all simple explanations" (Happé 2000, 203). Rather than attempt to explain all of the strengths and weaknesses inherent in autism via a single theory, it may be more fruitful to examine the ways in which the theories may work together, or complement each other. For example, it is possible to link all three of the above explanations of autism. There is some speculation that "autistic weakness in central coherence (could) be another facet of impaired executive function" (Frith 2003, 180); thus, these two theories may be entirely consistent with one another. Frith and Happé mention that executive function deficits may account for impaired theory of mind (Frith and Happé 1999, 9; Happé 2000, 215). Glüer and Pagin suggest, for example, that executive function disorders may result in a permanent block of appropriate theory of mind inferences, thereby rendering anyone with significant executive function blind to others' mentalizing. If weak central coherence is one aspect of weak executive function, and weak executive function accounts for the theory of mind deficits in autism, this does not dispute the theory of mind thesis, it merely further explains the source of theory of mind deficits.

The three competing theories may be compatible. O'Loughlin and Thagard discuss the possibility that a deficit in theory of mind accounts for the social deficits that characterize autism, but weak central coherence accounts for other cognitive difficulties persons with autism face. While seemingly an unparsimonious account of a single syndrome, this dual account carries two important lessons. First, it is the case that the theory of mind account and the weak central coherence account are compatible. Second, given the nature of syndromes—in which different individuals have different symptoms to different degrees— perhaps the more complex account is more explanatorily robust.

Frith contends that *all three theories* "implicate high-level cognitive processes that have something to do with self-consciousness" (Frith 2003, 208). The theory of mind thesis, weak central coherence thesis, and weak executive function thesis all result in an inability of the autistic person to mentalize—to make intentional state attributions—as a means of coming to understand others. Given that self-understanding is achieved, at least in part, via an understanding of others, and given that persons with autism lack the ability to make mental state attributions of others, a person with autism's understanding of his own consciousness is achieved fitfully, if at all, on Frith's account. While each of the theories may explain some characteristics of autism, together they share the common feature that self-reflection among those with autism is not tied to the reflection of the self in others. Glüer and Pagin note that some psychologists hold that theory of mind deficits are the primary cause of autism, whereas some claim it is the *precursors* to theory of mind that are the primary cause (Glüer and Pagin 2003). Debates continue as to which of these three theories is the best descriptor of autism; whether there is a causal connection among them; which of the deficits, if any, is causally prior; and how each of them interact (Happé 2000). Despite the continuing debate, Glüer and Pagin's discussion of autism and philosophy of language makes considerable use of this point: "For our purposes it is sufficient if [the theory of mind hypothesis] provides a *true description* of autistic behaviour and psychology. It does not have to be explanatory, much less provide the full explanation" (Glüer and Pagin 2003, 28).

Glüer and Pagin are correct. There is nothing in the competing accounts of autism that is incompatible with the *descriptive claims* made by the theory of mind theory. Perhaps other theories offer a causal explanation as to how persons with autism come to lack a functioning theory of mind, or perhaps theory of mind deficits can be cashed out in terms of weak executive function, or weak central coherence. John Lawson, for example, posits the Depth Accessibility Difficulties theory of autism in an attempt to bring together the theory of mind theory, weak executive function, weak central coherence, and the extreme male brain thesis into a single theory (Lawson 2003). One implication of Lawson's account is discussed in chapter 3. However, even if the weak executive function or weak central coherence theory is a more apt description of the *cause* of autism, this does not change the fact that persons with autism have tremendous difficulties recognizing the mental lives of others. Stuart Shanker (2004) postulates that the sensory difficulties that persons with autism experience lay the groundwork for some types of emotional detachment. Autism often results in extreme sensory sensitivity: bright lights, loud noises, or even scratchy clothing are reported by persons with autism as not merely annoying but as utterly excruciating. Shanker considers the possibility that infants with autism shy away from others, averting their gaze because of the stresses of eye contact. The result is that the child with autism "may not be able to comprehend the rules of complex social interactions or develop a sense of self . . . what later looks like a mind-reading deficit, therefore, may be the result of a dynamic process in which the child's lack of emotional interactions has intensified specific, early, sensory challenges and derailed the development of critical social, emotional, communicative, and cognitive capacities" (Shanker 2004, 227). Further implications of this view are explored in chapter 5. What is significant at this point is that sensory difficulties are postulated as causal explanation of theory of mind difficulties. Whether or not the sensory theory is a true causal explanation for theory of mind deficits, theory of mind problems persist. Even that small percentage of persons with autism who *do* pass theory of mind tests are often characterized as treating other persons in a more theory-based way than do non-autistic individuals (McGeer 2001). This labored way of coming to understand other people bespeaks an inability to understand others in the same way that non-autistic persons do. The evidence from false-belief tasks demonstrates this to be true, and while other accounts may point to global deficits that account for a lack of theory of mind, this does not change the fact that persons with autism can be described as having theory of mind deficiencies. Theory of mind deficiencies are undoubtedly intriguing from a psychological perspective. But they are also of tremendous interest from a philosophical perspective. The first of these philosophical complexities is autism's unique role in the theory theory versus simulation theory debate.

Autism's Challenge to Two Theories Explaining Human Behavior: Theory Theory and Simulation Theory

John is sitting alone in a room, reading. He gets up, walks to the window, closes the window, and sits back down. Marci watches him, and asks herself why John interrupted his concentration, only to sit back down.

One theory of explanation of human behavior is "folk psychology"—a belief/desire theory of explanation of human action. Folk psychology would explain John's behavior by ascribing intentional states such as the desire to be relieved of a draft, and his belief that closing the window would help—hence, folk psychology offers "intentional explanations" of human behavior. Folk psychology is not the only theory of explanation of human behavior, and it is highly contested. But even in the face of detractors, folk psychology persists, in part due to the intuitive, common-sense appeal of its belief/desire explanation of human actions. "In everyday life we make sense of each other's behavior by appeal to a belief-desire psychology" (Frith and Happé 1999, 2). In an attempt to strengthen the plausibility of folk psychology, is there anything that can be done to further elaborate on these intentional explanations of human behavior?

One way to present an even more robust folk psychological explanation is to elaborate on what is behind observers' intentional ascriptions. Marci might explain John's behavior by saying, "John wanted to feel warmer, and thought that the open window made the room too drafty, so he got up to close it." But what is behind Marci's claims that *John wanted*, or *John thought*, as a basis for explaining John's behavior? Two possibilities emerge.[5] The first is known as *theory theory*: observers theorize that the agents whose actions are being explained have a certain set of beliefs or desires—Marci ascribes to John a set of theories that explain his behavior. To do so, Marci must have a theory of mind. Furthermore, these intentions Marci ascribes to John may not be shared by Marci herself—perhaps she's quite comfortable, not at all bothered by the draft. But Marci, using a theory of mind, theorizes that John has a set of theories in the form of beliefs (if I close the window, the draft will go away) and desires (I want to feel warmer right about now). This theory of explanation behind John's getting up to close the window is a theory that postulates that John himself is theorizing, hence *theory theory* (TT). The individual who employs TT need not possess an elaborate theoretical mechanism behind intentional ascriptions; rather, the theory that is invoked is merely the postulating of mental events on the part of the agent whose behavior is explained. Similarly, people who use TT may be otherwise theory-deficient—the four-year-old child who uses TT to explain the behavior of others around him is no accomplished theorist, he is merely taking an intentional stance toward others (Gordon and Barker 1994).

A second possibility allows Marci to remain agnostic about John's intentions, but at the same time utilize a folk psychological explanation of his behavior. Rather than postulating a set of intentions on John's behalf, Marci asks herself what intentional states *she* would have were she in John's position, which if ascribed to John, would explain his behavior. After all, Marci does not have direct access to John's mental states, and to postulate an explanation of his behavior on the basis of intentions to which she has no direct access may be foolhardy. As John A. Barker states, this is one of the perils of folk psychology: it commits Marci to a "misconception-prone ontology," postulating the existence of intentions that she cannot know with certainty are actually there (Barker 2002, 34). But Marci does have direct access to her own mental states. Thus, she may simulate what it would be like to occupy John's situation, making use of the counterfactual "Were I sitting down in that room, only to get up, close the window and then sit back down, then I would have done so because I was cold and desired to suppress the draft." In this case, the explanation of John's behavior requires that Marci simulates a set of intentions on John's behalf, hence *simulation theory* (ST):

> According to the simulationist, folk-psychological interpretation of an individual's behavior is accomplished by means of "mental simulations" of the individual's decision-making situation. These pretense-like activities in which the cognitive system operates in a disengaged, or off-line manner, allegedly generate reliable predictions and explanations without need of a theory. (Barker 2002, 31)

ST is an alternative explanation of John's behavior that is open to Marci, in which she uses folk psychology without making intentional attributions that she cannot possibly know to be correct. Folk psychological explanations are preserved using ST, but no theory of mind needs to be postulated in order to generate these explanations.[6]

Which of these theories—TT or ST—is a true description of the intentional ascriptions behind folk psychological explanations?

Barker believes that ST is a better explanation, in part because it is simpler than TT. Occam's razor states "do not multiply entities beyond necessity"—do not postulate the existence of a more elaborate mechanism, or postulate the existence of more entities in the service of an explanation, when a simpler, less elaborate explanation will function just as well. Without direct access to John's mental states, Marci is left postulating the existence of mental states on John's part that may or may not exist. But with ST, she does not multiply those mental entities beyond necessity. Rather, she merely makes intentional ascriptions on her own behalf, still preserving folk psychology, but without making claims about intentions that she can never access directly. Using ST, Marci can "read John's mind," even as she is agnostic as to whether John has a mind to read, and agnostic about the intentions that abide in John's so-called mind. Proponents of this position cite the fact that TT requires Marci to possess a theory of mind when explaining John's actions, whereas ST does not require Marci to use a theory of mind. Thus ST is doubly parsimonious over TT: Marci need not ascribe intentional states or a mind to John, and no one need ascribe a theory of mind to Marci for ST to work.

A second advantage of ST over TT is that the inability of persons with autism to employ ST may provide an account of not only a failure of mindreading on the part of persons with autism, but also the lack of pretend play (Gordon and Barker 1994). Typically developing children who use ST would find pretend play to be a natural outgrowth of the simulation that they normally engage in so as to explain others' behavior. But persons with autism, who don't employ ST, would not easily take to imaginative play. Since a failure to use ST explains more of the deficits faced by persons with autism, proponents of ST believe that evidence from autism supports an ST account over a TT account.

One question that might emerge when considering ST is whether Marci needs to have access to her own intentions in order to run a successful simulation, or whether Marci can be as agnostic about her own intentional states as she is about the agent whose actions she attempts to explain. On one hand, Barker claims that the simulation theorist does not need "introspective ability or understanding of the self.... Nor need the mindreader employ any assumptions about what is transpiring—the entire simulation process can take place automatically, with no conscious awareness on the part of the simulator" (Barker 2002, 36). Here Barker claims that the simulator need not be aware of her own mental states. But later he asserts "To achieve reliability, the mindreader must attend to the propositions constituting the contents of the target individual's known beliefs and utilize these propositions in off-line inferences that roughly accord with the individual's own inferences" (Barker 2002, 40). The revised claim is that the simulator must be aware of her own inferences in order to successfully employ ST. Can one be aware of one's own inferences without being aware of one's own intentional states? It is unclear how simulation theory would work if Marci were not aware of her own intentional states. Furthermore, in order to genuinely suppress *her own* intentions, putting those intentions "off-line" in order to simulate John's intentions, Marci must be aware enough of her own intentions to be able to take them off-line. In other words, Marci needs to be aware of her own belief that she is not cold in order to then go off-line and simulate a response on the part of John, which includes as part of the explanation of his behavior that John would be cold. It does not seem plausible that Marci could put her own intentional states off-line if she did not recognize them herself. Thus, the claim that one of ST's advantages is that it does not require as great a level of self-reflection on the part of the individual postulating an explanation does not ring true. However, the claim that ST is simpler, because it does not require the postulating of intentional states on the part of other agents, agents whose intentional states are not directly available to the individual explaining that agent's actions, remains intact.

Shaun Nichols and Stephen Stich (2003) are proponents of TT and take issue with the claim that ST is simpler than TT.[7] Their argument is that postulating a theory of mind, which is required for TT, requires the same amount of conceptual work on the part of an agent as does ST. The two theories' method of explanation can be summarized using the following steps:

Theory Theory	Simulation Theory
1. Marci sees John close the window.	1. Marci sees John close the window.

2. Marci uses a *special database of psychological principles (theory of mind)* to explain why John closed the window.
3. Marci has an explanation for John's actions.

2. Marci goes "off-line," *using an off-line control mechanism,* to simulate why John closed the window.
3. Marci has an explanation for John's actions.

Is ST's step 2 really easier than TT's step 2? It would appear than both steps postulate equally complex maneuvers on the part of Marci: is there a simplicity advantage in having a theory of mind over an off-line control mechanism? "While the simulation theories get the database for free, it looks like the theory-theorist gets the 'control mechanism' for free" (Nichols and Stich 2003, 53). Philosophical arguments alone may not determine which of these two theories is the simpler.[8]

Regardless of the simplicity claims, step 2 in both TT and ST pose challenges for autistic agents. Since TT requires agents to make intentional ascriptions of others when explaining their behaviors, TT will work only for those who possess a theory of mind. If Marci has autism, using a TT explanation could prove difficult. Agents who have theory of mind deficiencies cannot use TT as a means of explaining the actions of other agents. ST, on the other hand, does not require agents to have a theory of mind, as the simulation theorist can remain agnostic about the intentional states of other agents. Thus, for autistic agents, ST may be available as an explanation of others' behavior in a way that TT is not.

But would ST really be that much easier for an autistic Marci? ST would require her to suppress her own propositional attitudes, using an off-line control mechanism, in order to explain John's behavior. Two problems emerge. The first concerns the ability for autistic agents to use an off-line control mechanism owing to difficulties that autistic persons have with imaginative play and other pretense-like behavior. Given that children with autism have difficulty with imaginative behaviors, such as pretend play, ST would be problematic, per Gordon and Barker (1994). ST requires agents to suppress their own intentional states so as to best simulate the intentional states of others. This would be difficult on a weak executive function hypothesis account, as a person with autism would be unable to suppress his own intentional states on the way toward simulating those of another agent. On the unified consciousness view simulation would be impossible—why would Marci take her own beliefs off-line and substitute them for John's beliefs, if Marci believed that John's beliefs were the same as her own? Daniel D. Hutto observes that ST is used within a context "in which the simulator is already aware that others will have different viewpoints" (Hutto 2003, 353)—a problem for both executive function theories and theory of mind theories of autism. Hutto cites the unified consciousness view as the reason that persons with autism are not able to offer narratives about others' lives: given a failure to appreciate that others have intentional states distinct from their own, persons with autism are unable to construct compelling explanations of human behavior. Elsewhere, Alvin Goldman (2006) similarly holds that three views of autism—the empathizing versus systematizing account, the weak executive functioning account, and the weak central coherence account—are all consistent with ST deficits. This lack of availability of ST is one way in which the weak executive function hypothesis and the theory of mind hypothesis both result in an inability for a person with autism to appreciate the propositional attitudes of other agents.

The second concern is that while ST does not appear at first glance to require mindreading, perhaps ST requires more theory of mind than it would first appear. TT requires Marci to make explicit intentional ascriptions of John. But ST requires Marci to make, at the very least, some type of indirect intentional ascriptions. As mentioned above, Barker makes clear that Marci must make use of her own inferences, even as she simulates the intentions of John in making sense of John's actions. Even as Marci puts many of her own propositional attitudes off-line (I don't believe that this room is cold; I don't want it to be warmer), and retains some of them in the form of simulations (If I were bothered by the draft, I would close the window), she also ascribes propositional attitudes to John (John always wants it to be warmer; John believes that if you sit near an open window that you'll catch a cold). To say that one can successfully use ST without a theory of mind is mistaken. For this reason, Hutto believes that "simulation approaches should be classified as a sub-species of theory-theory" (Hutto 2003, 352). Diana Raffman holds that "the evidence from autism is neutral; it favors neither position [TT or ST] over the other" (Raffman 1999, 30). Both TT and ST are problematic for persons with autism; the evidence from autism is no reason to prefer one theory over the other. The upshot is that two of the most prominent theories that further elaborate on folk psychological explanations—TT and ST—pose considerable difficulties for autistic agents. TT explicitly requires agents to have a theory of mind, while ST is problematic for persons with autism due both to its commitment to pretense, as well as its less explicit commitment to theory of mind.

In summary, TT and ST are alternative ways of expounding on the folk psychological explanation of human behavior, but both are problematic for autistic agents. Autism does not provide evidence for choosing either TT or ST over the other. However, the inapplicability of either TT or ST for autistic agents has interesting ethical implications. Understanding other agents, and understanding others' agency, is of significance in ethics: an understanding of others is invaluable when learning to become a morally responsible agent. Victoria Mc-Geer observes that explanations of human behavior are commonly tied to normative evaluations—our expectations about what individuals *actually* do, what they are *expected* to do, and what they *ought* to do are all tied together (McGeer 2001). As important as understanding others, however, is understanding ourselves. Thus, the next topic of consideration is the challenge that autism poses for philosophical theories of self-consciousness.

Autism and Self-Consciousness

Is it the case, for example, that we are first aware of our own mental states, and that we then extend this experience to others by analogy ... ? ... However, it is hard to understand why, if this first-person experience is so important, children with autism fail to develop a normal mindreading system, since they presumably experience mental states themselves. An alternative position ... is that we not only have these mental states but we are able to introspect on them, and that it is the knowledge that is a product of such introspection that we ascribe to others. This position seems plausible, since this would then

predict that both introspection and ascription of mental states to others would be hard for children with autism. There is some evidence
that this is the case. (Baron-Cohen 1995, 130)

If persons with autism have difficulty ascribing mental states to
others, might they also have difficulty ascribing mental states to themselves? The claim is not that persons with autism fail to have mental
states, but rather, that they lack awareness of their own mental states.
The failure of introspection that Baron-Cohen suggests above would
challenge some philosophical conceptions of what it is to hold a particular propositional attitude. Typically, when it is said of an agent A
that A *believes P*, it is also true that A *believes that A believes P*. Agents are
expected to have epistemic access to their own mental states in a way
that is not true of other facts about the world: A's belief that A *believes*
that P is more easily justified, in many cases simply by virtue of the
fact that A believes it, whereas A can be mistaken about his belief that
some other agent, B, believes that P. Raffman points out that the picture
is not always as clear as this, owing to tacit beliefs, or unconscious
mental activities. Even in the face of such confounding factors, the
view that we have direct access to our own minds persists:

> To be sure, certain elements of the Cartesian view are retained—in
> particular the idea that we occupy a privileged epistemic position in
> respect of the contents of our own *conscious occurrent* states (perhaps
> especially our occurrent sensations). The assumption is that we nor-
> mally have better access to our own conscious occurrent states than
> others do. (This idea is often expressed by saying that we enjoy *first*
> *person authority* with respect to these states.) Nevertheless, the
> possibility of error is always open. (Raffman 1999, 25)

The fact that agents typically have access to the content of their own
minds, and yet they can also make mistakes, demonstrates that access
to our own propositional attitudes is what Raffman calls a *cognitive*
achievement. In saying that this is a *cognitive achievement*, it is acknowl-
edged that agents can be mistaken, and thus some sort of justification
is necessary in order to say that one has knowledge of the content of
one's own mind. This view is contrasted with infallibilism—the view
that we cannot be wrong about the content of our own mental states.

If it is possible to be wrong about our sensory experiences (is the light green or blue?) or it is possible to be wrong about intentional self-ascriptions (do I believe that Lee can be trusted?) then some means must exist that enable this to occur. What is the mechanism by which this achievement is realized? A theory of mind is essential for agents to attribute beliefs to others. Might the same mechanism by which we attribute beliefs to *others* be the mechanism by which we attribute beliefs to *ourselves*? If so, then a person who is deficient with respect to theory of mind may not be aware of his own mental states. This is not to say that the person who lacked a theory of mind did not *have* mental states; rather, the person with a compromised theory of mind would be unable to reflect on his own mental states:

> The logical extension of the [theory of mind] deficit account of autism is that individuals with autism may know as little about their own minds as about the minds of other people. This is not to say that these individuals lack mental states, but that in an important sense they are unable to reflect on their mental states. Simply put, they lack the cognitive machinery to represent their thoughts and feelings *as* thoughts and feelings. (Frith and Happé 1999, 7)

Frith and Happé concede that this idea is "one that we have shied away from, since it seemed potentially pernicious to attribute impaired self-consciousness to those who are handicapped and not able to present their own side of things" (Frith and Happé 1999, 1–2).[9] Additionally, higher-functioning persons with autism appear to have a degree of self-consciousness in proportion to their ability to pass false-belief tests and other indicators of theory of mind. But for those individuals with impaired theory of mind, questions about their level of self-consciousness persist.

An intriguing psychological test lends support to the claim that persons with autism have difficulty introspecting on their own intentional states. In the test, children are given a toy gun and a set of targets, and asked to state their intended target. The outcome of the shot is then manipulated, so that in some cases the child hits the originally stated target, and in some cases, the child "misses." When asked "Which one did you mean to hit?" typically developing four-year-olds answer the question correctly, "but children with autism often made the error of answering by reference to the actual outcome" (Baron-Cohen 2000b, 11; Phillips, et al. 1998). Children with autism have difficulty reporting on what they believed that they believed. This experiment is taken to demonstrate that children with autism have difficulty reflecting on their own thoughts. While the theory of mind thesis, the weak central coherence thesis, and the weak executive function thesis all offer equally plausible accounts of this failure of introspection, the result is the same—children with autism do not demonstrate an ability to introspect their own intentional states. Perner and Lang (2000) discuss the theory that the self-monitoring that is only possible with an intact theory of mind is required for the impulse control that typifies executive function. Thus, a causal relation between theory of mind and weak executive function is revealed when the question of self-consciousness is explored: a failure of theory of mind results in failure of self-consciousness, which in turn results in weak executive function.

Successful application of ST requires a certain level of self-awareness. "All the versions of simulation rely on the idea that I can predict your behaviour by extrapolating from my own mind" (Gopnik et al. 2000, 59). The agent who employs ST must be sufficiently aware of her mental states so as to first put them off-line, second pick out the relevant propositional attitude from a counterfactual (If I were in that cold room, then I would *want to quell the draft* by closing the window), and third ascribe that propositional attitude to another agent as a way of explaining that other agent's actions. As mentioned above, if Marci were not aware of her own mental states, she would not be able to successfully put them off-line so that she could then determine what John would do, given his mental states. Thus, the question of self-consciousness has implications for the TT and ST debate.[10]

Frith and Happé's argument about the lack of self-consciousness of the part of persons with autism rests on the claim that the mechanism by which agents come to learn about the mental states of others is the same mechanism by which agents come to learn about their own mental states. Thus autistic agents "know what is transpiring in their own minds only by applying an explicit theory of mind to their own behaviour" (Raffman 1999, 23). Frith and Happé present three pieces of evidence in favor of the claim that these two mechanisms are one and the same. First, the literature on human development indicates that agents do not attribute a given mental state to others before those agents are able to attribute that mental state to themselves. Second, when agents are unable to attribute certain mental states to others, they do not attribute those mental states to themselves either (Frith and Happé 1999). Third, they cite self-reports from persons with autism which they believe demonstrate a lack of self-consciousness of their own mental states.

Nichols and Stich consider the claim that TT does not merely offer an explanation of others' mental states, but that it also offers an agent an explanation of his own mental states: "The core idea of the TT account of self-awareness is that the process of reading one's own mind is largely or entirely parallel to the process of reading someone else's mind" (Nichols and Stich 2003, 163). And why should it not be? If the way agents come to understand other intentional agents is by attributing theories to them, it only stands to reason that agents then come to understand themselves by attributing theories to themselves (Gopnik, et al. 2000). Or perhaps, agents come to understand themselves as intentional agents first, and then come to recognize a similarity between themselves and other agents. In this case, the agent applies the same theories to others as he first applied to himself. In either case, however, the agent uses TT, which implies a theory of mind, to understand both himself and others.

The implications of a lack of introspective ability become more significant when the link between consciousness and self-consciousness is examined. What is it for an agent to be conscious, if that agent is not conscious of his consciousness? Sartre, for example, believed that consciousness was always consciousness of *something*, and unless it is possible for an agent to be conscious of his consciousness in a full-blown sense, that agent could not be said to be conscious at all. Thus, a lack of introspection on the part of the person who lacks a theory of mind raises even more significant questions about the very consciousness of that person.

Raffman disputes the conclusion that people come to know their own minds in the same way that they come to know the minds of others, via an explicit theory of mind. Most of the evidence from self-reports of persons with Asperger's syndrome does not indicate that persons with autism lack self-awareness in the sense that they fail to have propositional attitudes, but that they lack the *concepts* that someone who was fluent in the language of the mind needs in order to conceptualize intentional states—a position Raffman refers to as the "Conceptual Incompetence" hypothesis (Raffman 1999, 24). The conclusion that the mechanism by which we learn to understand ourselves and the mechanism by which we learn to understand others is one and the same is too hasty. If there are distinct mechanisms by which people come to understand their own propositional attitudes, and the mental states of others, then it is possible that while autistic agents have difficulty coming to understand others' minds, they may nonetheless have an understanding of their own minds.

McGeer finds TT to be an inadequate means by which agents come to know themselves. TT is so theory-laden as to effectively make the agent an object of his own study, making the agent alien to himself. Theoretical expertise, she argues, "does not generally produce such feelings of attunement between the knower and the objects known, even when the objects know are (in some sense) ourselves" (McGeer 2001, 116). Theoretical expertise remains the expertise of "an outside observer looking on," and thus does not illuminate "seeing in other people *our own ways of being*" (McGeer 2001, 116). Elsewhere, McGeer (2004) argues that Frith and Happé's discussion of autistic persons' self-reports does not evidence a lack of introspective self-awareness. The mistake, McGeer argues, is that Frith and Happé rely too heavily on a Cartesian "neoperceptual model, [that] we are self-conscious to the extent that we are able to access or track the first-order states and processes that constitute the real bedrock of our mental lives—our beliefs, desires, perceptual experiences, and so forth" (McGeer 2004, 243).[11] On this neoperceptual model, we then make reports about these mental states based on second-order judgments about them. McGeer's objection to this model is that the knowledge one would need in order to accomplish these second-order accounts requires the formation of "third-order states that reflect subjects' knowledge of their contents" (McGeer 2004, 245). The problem here is not so much an infinite regress, but that it renders the self-reports of persons with autism conceptually incoherent. An autistic person would have first-order mental states, *would not* have the second-order judgments required to adequately capture those first-order mental states, but *would* have the *third-order* mechanism needed to *adequately fail* to capture their second-order mental states. "For instance, autistics are presumed to give adequate linguistic expressions to their inadequate sensory awareness of their normal sensory experience" (McGeer 2004, 245). For this reason, McGeer abandons the neoperceptual model in favor of a "direct expressivist model of self-awareness," in which a person's self-report of both sensory experience and intentional states simply *are* the individual's sensory experiences or intentional states. Elsewhere, McGeer calls this a reflective expressivist model (McGeer 2005). On one hand, such a position accepts infallibilism. Some may see this as a weakness (Goldman 2006, 225); McGeer sees it as a strength. Why should we not be infallible about our occurrent sensations? On the other hand, the model "will enable us to construe autistic reports as detailed expressions of abnormal models of experience, not as inaccurate quasi-perceptual reports of normal modes of experience" (McGeer 2004, 249)—in McGeer's estimation, an unabashed strength.

Nichols and Stich ultimately reject TT as a means of coming to understand *our own* mental states, even though TT can be used successfully to attribute mental states to others. Rather, they claim that agents posses a self-monitoring mechanism (MM) which agent use to monitor their own propositional attitudes, as well as theory of mind, a separate mechanism, which agents use to explain others' behavior via propositional attitude ascription. In their estimation, "when normal adults believe that p, they can quickly and accurately form the belief *I believe that p;* when normal adults desire that p, they can quickly and accurately form the belief *I desire that p;* and so on for the rest of the propositional attitudes. In order to implement this ability, no sophisticated [theory of mind] is required" (Nichols and Stich 2003, 170). The speed and accuracy with which agents self-identify intentional states contributes to the likelihood that the means by which we make these self-ascriptions is via a dedicated mechanism, MM. The fact that intentional attribution to others is less accurate than self-attribution supports the claim that a separate mechanism is utilized. In postulating MM in addition to theory of mind, Nichols and Stich, *contra* Mc-Geer, deny that understanding other agents is essential to understanding ourselves. Furthermore, they claim that the empirical evidence, based on self-reports of persons with autism, demonstrates that some high-functioning persons with autism, such as some with Asperger's syndrome, do have self-awareness of their own mental states.

One ethical question that might emerge from the discussion of autism and self-consciousness concerns theories of personhood and well-lived human lives that emphasize consciousness, as well as self-consciousness. If consciousness and self-consciousness are essential to personhood, or to a well-lived human life, and a theory of mind is essential to self-consciousness, then the individual who lacks a theory of mind could be excluded from those categories. As shown in chapter 2, several such theories make use of consciousness and self-consciousness. Frith and Happé are right to warn against the pernicious results of the claim that some persons lack self-consciousness, given the significance that philosophers have accorded these properties.

Another concern that emerges from the discussion of the self-consciousness of persons with autism is that persons who do not have autism, and who are aware of their own conscious occurrent states, *cannot imagine what it would be like to not have direct access to their own mental states.* Individuals who have direct access to their propositional attitudes simply take for granted that *in believing P* they have an awareness they *believe that they believe P.* Individuals who have direct awareness of their conscious states might not be able to conceive of not having that access, and thus might not be able to conceive of what it would be like to be autistic. The gulf between persons with autism and those without autism seems wider and wider when it becomes clear that persons with autism cannot understand those without autism, and those without autism cannot understand what it would be like to have autism. McGeer puts it well when she says "we must be sure that however we specify what is lacking in autistic individuals, it explains our inability to get them as much as it explains their inability to get us" (McGeer 2001, 116). One of the lessons learned when examining the philosophical implications of autism and self-consciousness is that autistic and non-autistic persons may be living even more separate lives than previously imagined.

Autism and Philosophy of Language: Meaning Theories and Theory of Mind

One of the persistent questions in philosophy of language concerns the meaning of utterances. When speakers use language, what do they mean? And when hearers hear utterances, what do they think is meant by those utterances? Broadly speaking, there are two different accounts of what it is for an utterance to mean something. One type of theory uses an approach called the "theory of communication-intention" (Strawson 1970); such theories take "sentence-meaning as dependent on speakers-meaning, thus making the philosophy of mind and theory of speakers' intentions foundational for the philosophy of language," including Paul Grice's theory of non-natural meaning (Evnine 1991, 74). A second type of theory is one that stresses formal semantics, such as Donald Davidson's meaning theory. Davidson's theory embraces the view that "how mental states get their contents, and how sentences get their meanings, are interdependent" (Evnine 1991, 74). Despite their differences, Grice's and Davidson's theories are both challenged by the notion of autistic speakers who both have language competency and fail theory of mind tasks. Each of these philosophers' meaning theories is challenged in slightly different ways by the autistic language user.

Persons with autism who are unable to use language are not counterexamples to any theory of meaning. Nor are persons with autism who are competent language users, and who pass false-belief tasks, counterexamples to the theories presented here. Since most false-belief tasks require a high level of language ability, the very fact that someone can be said to have failed a false-belief task, in any interesting sense, requires that he must also have language competency. Language competency can contribute to an understanding of false beliefs and other aspects of theory of mind (Tager-Flusberg and Joseph 2005), allowing some persons with autism to pass false-belief tasks. However, individuals who *both* fail false-belief tasks, thereby calling into question their theory of mind, *and* have language competency pose difficulties for the meaning theories discussed here.

Persons with autism who fail false-belief tasks and yet nonetheless use language often have difficulties in many aspects of language use, such as understanding sarcasm, irony, and pragmatics in general. These aspects of language use are particularly tied to theory of mind[12] as they require speakers to be aware of others' roles in language use: "Almost every aspect of pragmatics involves sensitivity to speaker and listener mental states, and hence mindreading, though it is important to note that pragmatics also involves using context" (Baron-Cohen 2000b, 13). For this reason, Baron-Cohen says that either theory of mind deficits or weak central coherence could contribute to difficulties in pragmatics for autistic speakers.

Happé reviews studies that show that persons with autism fare just as well recalling lists of unconnected words as they do recalling words that are linked by either semantic relations or by grammatical relations (Happé 2000, 210). This is counter-intuitive for most language users—the words "lion, tiger, cougar, puma, cheetah, jaguar" are easier to remember than "lion, wheelbarrow, enigma, grease, harrow, fork," precisely because the meaning of the first six words are linked, whereas the meanings of the second list of words has no immediate connection.[13] If autistic language users find both lists just as easy, or just as difficult, to recall, this may demonstrate that meaning does not *mean* for the autistic speaker what it means for the non-autistic speaker. Thus, there may be some empirical basis for demonstrating that persons with autism may appear to be language users, but do not mean by their words what non-autistic language users mean. The first of two meaning theories challenged by the autistic language user is Grice's.

Paul Grice's Account of Non-Natural Meaning

Grice distinguished the meaning of utterances, which have "non-natural meaning," or meaning$_{nn}$, with "natural meaning," the meaning that allows us to conclude that if winter comes, that *means* spring cannot be far behind. Meaning$_{nn}$ requires speakers to have beliefs about their utterances, and the effects of those utterances on the beliefs of hearers. A speaker means$_{nn}$ something by an utterance if and only if the speaker intends, in making that utterance, "to produce some effect in an audience by means of the recognition of this intention," namely, to produce the effect (Grice 1957, 385). According to Grice's account of meaning$_{nn}$, speakers must have a fourth-order intention, as represented by the following account of what it is for speaker S to *mean P* when S says utterance u to a hearer H:

> when uttering u, S intends for H to believe that S intends for H to believe that P

Perhaps S *believes P*: this is a *first-order* intention (there is a single intentional ascription). If S *intends* for H to *believe P*, then this would describe a *second-order* intention on S's part. The Gricean account of meaning$_{nn}$ involves a fourth-order intention. When S says to H "It is cold with the window open," S's utterance is meaningful if and only if, in uttering u, S intends for H to believe something, and in particular, S intends for H to believe that S intended for H to believe that it is cold with the window open.

The Gricean account of meaning$_{nn}$ does not commit speakers to explicitly have these fourth-order intentions, but on reflection they must recognize that these intentions are behind their utterances. For the individual with a compromised theory of mind who is unable to pass false-belief tasks, this theory of meaning presents unique problems. The speaker who is unable to attribute false-beliefs to his hearer may also be unable to attribute any type of belief to his hearer: recall Glüer and Pagin's observation that "to understand the difference between *being* true and being *believed* to be true, one must understand that a belief can be false, and this understanding is manifested by means of the ability to ascribe beliefs one takes to be false" (Glüer and Pagin 2003, 27). Understanding the concept of "belief" requires the understanding of the concept of a "false belief." If this is the case, then the autistic speaker cannot have fourth-order intentions about his utterance, not even the implicit fourth-order intentions needed for the utterance to have any meaning at all:

> Of course, the Gricean account does not require the speaker to attribute a false belief to the hearer, only intend the hearer to have a (possibly so far unpossessed) belief. But, to repeat, the problem is *not* that

> there is only a problem with attributing *false* beliefs. The problem is
> that understanding what it is to have a false belief is an essential part
> of understanding what it is to have a belief at all. (Glüer and Pagin
> 2003, 37)

Even those individuals with autism who are able to pass first-order false-belief tasks are often unable to pass second- and higher-order false-belief tasks. The fourth-order intentionality required to mean$_{nn}$ something on Grice's view is beyond the ability of most autistic speakers. The evidence from competent autistic speakers demonstrates that Grice's theory of meaning is incorrect. A theory of meaning that requires speakers to have fourth-order intentions precludes the possibility of competent speakers who do not have a theory of mind. But since such speakers exist—autistic speakers who are both competent in language and who do not have a theory of mind—this theory of meaning must be incorrect. Another candidate for a plausible meaning theory must be found.

David Lewis attempts to elaborate on Grice's account demonstrating that meaning$_{nn}$ is tied to linguistic *conventions*—"meaning$_{nn}$ is a consequence of conventional signaling" (Lewis 1969, 154). Conventions make use of what is held to be *common knowledge* in a population (Lewis 1969). On Lewis's account, both common knowledge and conventions make significant use of intentions, which are confounding to the individual whose theory of mind is compromised. For example, Lewis presents the following analysis of "common knowledge":

> Let us say that it is *common knowledge* in a population P that _____
> if and only if some state of affairs A holds such that:
>
> (1) Everyone in P has reason to believe that A holds,
> (2) A indicates to everyone in P that everyone in P has reason to
>   believe that A holds,
> (3) A indicates to everyone in P that _____. (Lewis 1969, 56)

Lewis elaborates that *agreement, salience,* and *precedents* are all important to a population's basis for common knowledge (Lewis 1969, 57).[14] The implications for someone who is lacking a theory of mind is clear. A compromised theory of mind can lead to questions as to what counts as a knowledge condition (Baron-Cohen 1995), calling into question

(1), above. Thus, (2) is also called into question, as persons with autism may not know what counts as an indicator to everyone in *P* that they have reason to believe *A*. While *A* may indicate to everyone in *P* that _____ , without (1) and (2), the autistic person does not have reason to believe *A*. Finally, in addition to the knowledge conditions for *A* being problematic, the fact that common knowledge is about the *recognition that other agents have a set of beliefs* is also problematic for autistic agents. Thus, failures of theory of mind prevent the autistic speaker from holding common knowledge with the rest of the population. Since, for Lewis, common knowledge is an essential part of the conventions of a population, it follows that the person lacking a theory of mind cannot be said to follow the conventions of the population: "Higher-order expectations are the heart of conventions. And higher-order expectations are what our proposed autistic speakers lack" (Glüer and Pagin 2003, 42). Thus, an account of meaning in terms of linguistic conventions is similarly unavailable to the autistic speaker.

Lewis may have anticipated this point, as indicated by the following:

> Consider the conventions of a language, whatever they may be. Anyone who is a member of a population *P*, and party to its conventions of language, must know what those conventions are. If any regularity *R* is in fact a convention of language in *P*, any normal member of *P* must have reason to believe that *R* satisfies the defining conditions for a convention. (Lewis 1969, 62)

Lewis includes a footnote here, elaborating on the term "normal": "Not counting children and the feeble-minded, who may conform to *R* without expecting conformity and without preferring to conform conditionally upon the conformity of others" (Lewis 1969, 62, n.1). Leaving aside objectionable language on Lewis's part, his point is that there are some persons who may not share common knowledge of the conventions of the language, and as such, are not party to that language's conventions. Glüer and Pagin observe, "It might be objected that convention does not require that each and every member of a community has the required higher-order thought capacities. Some members could be allowed a kind of parasitic membership, while core members would still need the capacities" (Glüer and Pagin 2003, 43, n.29). What status is left to those persons who do not have common knowledge, either because they are being initiated into the conventions of the language, or, like the person who lacks a theory of mind, will *never* be able to share common knowledge with the rest of the population?

Grice's theory requires speakers to have fourth-order intentions, a condition well beyond the abilities of individuals who lack a theory of mind. Lewis's attempts to elaborate on Gricean meaning$_{nn}$ by introducing the notions of convention and common knowledge do not rescue the theory for autistic speakers. Another theory of meaning needs to be found that is sufficiently inclusive.

Donald Davidson's Theory of Radical Interpretation

Davidson does not offer an account of meaning in terms of belief on the part of speakers, because in his estimation, belief and meaning are interdependent. To give an account of meaning in terms of beliefs would then assume that beliefs have causal priority. Instead, Davidson's account of meaning begins with the conditions under which a given sentence is true (Andrews 2002). "To know the meaning of a sentence one must know its truth conditions, to know how the world must be if the sentence is to be true" (Evnine 1991, 81). The truth conditions for a sentence are what give that sentence meaning. Davidson adopts Tarski's theory of truth (Tarski 1956): a given sentence, s, in the object language, L, is said to be true if and only if sentence p in the metalanguage L' provides the conditions under which s is true. The biconditional "s is true if and only if p" is a Tarskian T-sentence—once the biconditional in convention T is satisfied, then it can be said that a sentence s in language L is true by showing that p in the metalanguage L' is true. "Convention T requires that p be a translation of the sentence named by s" (Ramberg 1989, 57). Tarski's theory does not admit of the possibility that truth is relative to a given language, or a given speaker. The "sameness" of truth across speakers is essential in establishing Davidson's model of interpretation.

All speakers are interpreters of other speakers (Davidson 1984a). Speakers interpret the utterances of other speakers, with the expectation that what speakers say will be true. In this way all speakers undergo a process of *radical interpretation,* interpreting each others' utterances, and interpreting each of a speaker's utterances in the context of each of that speakers' other utterances. Radical interpretation is undertaken by employing Davidson's *principle of charity,* the principle that speakers typically say things that are true, and their utterances should be interpreted charitably with the expectation that those utterances are true. Speakers of any language are assumed to be saying things that are true and their beliefs are assumed to be non-contradictory. The principle of charity guards against attributing to speakers inexplicitly held beliefs, or beliefs that a speaker appears to have but which are unjustified. Eventually, the speaker and the hearer come to interpret one another by applying the principle of charity with an eye toward preserving the truthfulness of each others' utterances, and come to establish meaning of each others' utterances on this basis:

> [B]eliefs and meanings conspire to account for utterances. A speaker who holds a sentence to be true on an occasion does so in part because of what he means, or would mean, by an utterance of that sentence, and in part because of what he believes. (Davidson 1984a, 142)

In summary, each interpreter of others' utterances uses the principle of charity to radically interpret sentences in such a way that speakers can be interpreted as saying things that are true.

Evnine observes that along with attributing beliefs to individuals, part of Davidson's meaning theory is that interpreters must be able to attribute false beliefs to others. It is possible for speakers to be in error about their own beliefs, and interpreters must be able to recognize the false beliefs of speakers in order to correctly interpret what speakers are saying. On this account, to have the concept of a belief is also to have a concept of a false belief, otherwise there is no point in having, or attributing, beliefs at all (Andrews 2002, 320). Evidence from additional speakers, additional utterances by the same speaker, as well as convention T, can lead an interpreter to conclude that a speaker holds false or true beliefs. The mutual interpreters use the principle of charity, as well as convention T, in order to attribute meaning to each other. The truth conditions of sentences, as well as their meaning, are constituted by the states of affairs that make those sentences true. Thus, three parts of the Davidsonian triangle—speaker, interpreter, and the conditions that make sentences true—together provide the conditions that make words meaningful.

For autistic speakers, difficulties emerge when attempting to employ both radical interpretation as well as the principle of charity so as to interpret speakers' utterances. Radical interpretation, and hence meaning itself, requires users of language to make significant use of others' beliefs:

> Meaning, in the special sense in which we are interested when we talk of what an utterance literally means, gets its life from those situations in which someone intends (or assumes or expects) that his words will be understood in a certain way, and they are. In such cases we can say without hesitation: how he intended to be understood, and was understood, is what he, and his words, literally meant on that occasion. (Davidson 2005, 120)

Without a theory of mind, radical interpretation is impossible; without the ability to successfully attribute false beliefs, as well as true beliefs, the principle of charity is of no use. Radical interpretation is possible only if the interpreter ascribes intentionality to the speaker. "Indeed, the Principle of Charity could be taken as the skeleton of the theory of folk psychology" (Evnine 1991, 112). Given that there are some competent language users who fail to have a theory of mind, these speakers pose a counterexample to Davidson's meaning theory.

Glüer and Pagin argue that Davidson's radical interpretation and principle of charity are not challenged by autistic language users. On one hand, they concede that "an autistic speaker who fails theory of mind tests, and presumably lacks a capacity for higher-order thoughts, could not engage in methodologically proper radical interpretation. Applying the principle of charity explicitly involves judging the reasonableness of beliefs, which does require higher-order thought capacity" (Glüer and Pagin 2003, 44). However, Glüer and Pagin believe that autistic speakers are not counterexamples to Davidson's account, as "Neither Davidson's theory of the form of an explicit meaning theory about a speaker or a language, nor the principles he proposes for proper radical interpretation, are intended as providing a psychological model of actual interpreters" (Glüer and Pagin 2003, 45). Hanni Bouma makes a similar point, arguing that Davidson's theory is not vulnerable to empirical counterexamples, such as autistic speakers who both lack a theory of mind and yet are competent interpreters of other speakers (Bouma 2006a). This may be correct, but it is not clear that this point is sufficient to rescue Davidson's theory. Davidson did not set out to provide a psychological model of interpreters—the ability to attribute higher-order thought is not something that is *meant to follow* from the fact that persons are language users. Rather, according to Davidson, this is a pre-condition for being a language user. The interdependence of belief and language on his account shows that neither has causal priority, but one cannot exist without the other.

Glüer and Pagin make one more attempt to rescue Davidson's meaning theory in the face of the counterexample provided by autistic speakers. Autistic speakers "interpret in accordance with charity, together with the assumption that their interpretation is pretty mechanic and stereotypical, indicat[ing] that when it comes to language learning the autistic learner simply, automatically and permanently accepts everything the teacher says" (Glüer and Pagin 2003, 46). Perhaps autistic speakers are interpreters, but they do not do the actual work of interpreting themselves. Autistic speakers may be akin to individuals who are first learning a language, who may not be competent interpreters but whose utterances still have meaning. They may not fully use the principle of charity, but they are still language users. Does this rescue Davidson's theory? Andrews does not believe so. Andrews asks if autistic individuals can be compared to children, whose utterances appear meaningful, "because we believe that the child will at some point become a full participant in the [Davidsonian] triangle" (Andrews 2002, 320). The potential to enter into radical interpretation allows less-than-competent interpreters' utterances to be meaningful, as they make their way into full language proficiency. The problem, however, is that the autistic individual who lacks a theory of mind will not eventually make his way into that triangle, and thus will never be a competent language user. Andrews thus concludes that Davidson's meaning theory cannot accommodate competent language users who have autism, thereby showing Davidson's theory to be mistaken.

Bouma attempts to rescue Davidson's meaning theory. She presents a two-pronged attack on Kristin Andrews's (2002) contention that Davidson's theory is challenged by autistic speakers who lack a theory of mind. First, she argues that the empirical evidence of the lack of theory of mind on the part of persons with autism is at best mixed. Second, as previously stated, she holds that Davidson's theory is "not vulnerable to empirical counterexamples" (Bouma 2006b, 639). This is because the principle of charity is analytic in Davidson's schema—it is "constitutive of concepts such as belief, desire, and intention" (Bouma 2006b, 659). As such, the principle of charity is not vulnerable to empirical disconfirmation, including any supposed disconfirmation in the form of autistic language users. Andrews and Ljiljana Radenovic reply that the clinical evidence may in fact demonstrate that there are autistic language users who are not interpreters, and present a dialogue between an autistic schoolchild and his therapist which, in their estimation, demonstrates this point (Andrews and Radenovic 2006). Bouma responds that the transcript of the conversation cited actually proves that the autistic schoolboy is a much more sophisticated interpreter than Andrews and Radenovic claim (Bouma 2006a). Even when an autistic language user gets an answer wrong to a question about others' reasons for acting— in some cases horribly wrong—autistic language users still know what counts as a *reason*. They still use connectives or "sentences which are indexicals" (sentences which may be true in one context but false in another) correctly (Bouma 2006a, 681). This should be enough to demonstrate that they are interpreters, using language on Davidson's terms. But it is not clear that Bouma has done enough to show that autistic speakers are not akin to "parasitic" interpreters, as coined by Glüer and Pagin. The question that Bouma has left unanswered is whether autistic speakers could be radical interpreters of *each other's* speech, akin to those who are making their way toward language proficiency.[15] The contested evidence cited by Bouma, and Andrews and Radenovic concerns an exchange between an autistic boy and his non-autistic therapist. What might the Davidsonian triangle containing only autistic individuals tell us about language use?

There are of course other meaning theories besides the ones mentioned here. However, it is interesting to see how autism challenges two of the best-known theories, owing to the existence of competent autistic language users who nonetheless lack a theory of mind. Several ethical questions arise when considering that autistic speakers seem to be meaning something by their utterances, and yet some prominent theories cannot account for this. Communication—in whatever form—is often cited as part of what makes a human life uniquely human, but without language, it is hard to know how this is accomplished. Language is often an essential part of community and culture. Finally, if autistic and non-autistic people are operating using different meaning theories, the possibility persists that the two populations are—literally—talking past each other when attempting to resolve ethical dilemmas. The ethical implications of this divide become clearer in future chapters.

Autism and Modularity of Mind: Theory of Mind, Mental Modules, and the Ontology of Autism

Plato recounts an anecdote in the *Republic* about Leontius, who sees an executioner surrounded by corpses outside the city walls (Plato 1974, 439e–440a). On one hand, he is repulsed by the scene and is inclined to look away. On the other hand, he is captivated and cannot help but look. Finally, Leontius is overcome and moves toward the corpses saying of his eyes, "Look for yourselves, you evil things, get your fill of the beautiful sight" (Plato 1974, 440a). The lesson Plato takes away from this familiar story is that the soul/psyche/mind has several parts. One part may cause a man to turn away from the revolting scene, whereas another compels him to look. More than two thousand years ago, philosophers were attracted by the notion that the mind is not merely a homogeneous "thinking thing," but that the activities of the mind were separate and unique, that it was possible to distinguish between the many subsystems that characterized that thinking thing. Questions persist: What does it mean to be a *part* of a mind? What exactly *are* the different parts of the mind?

In his *The Modularity of Mind*, Jerry Fodor argues that the mind's subsystems are modular. Modular components of the mind receive input and send output, functioning in a relatively autonomous fashion. One example of a mental activity that is modular in nature is perception, another is language ability. Fodor contrasts these modular subsystems with those that are part of the mind's central processes. Scientific confirmation, for example, would not be a modular process (Fodor 1983, 104), even though the process of scientific confirmation is not possible without certain modular processes. Input systems such as perception are modular (Fodor 1983, 46).

Several questions arise when considering modularity and autism. First, is theory of mind a modular process or not? Second, what does the possibility that theory of mind is *not* modular tell us about the nature of autism? A third question that arises from the modularity debate concerns the nature of spectrum conditions, such as autism: is there any such thing as a *single disorder,* autism? To answer these questions, modularity must be better understood.

Modular subsystems have the following nine properties:[16]

(1) *Domain specificity:* Each module undertakes specific activities—there are "specialized systems for specialized tasks" (Fodor 1983, 52). For example, human speech is regulated by a domain specific aspect of the mind, as is visual perception;

(2) *Mandatoriness:* Agents do not have a choice to interpret input, or accept input; Fodor holds that the input from modules is mandatory. Objects appear to our visual perception whether we want them to or not; we don't have any choice but to understand words uttered in our native language, even when we would prefer not to hear the words as words (Fodor 1983, 53);

(3) *Lack of central access to the mental representations of modules:* Agents are aware of the input that is fed into modules, and the output generated by the modules, but not the intermediate mental representations that occur between initial input and the final output. "The subject doesn't have equal access to all of these ascending levels of representation" (Fodor 1983, 56);

(4) *Speed:* Modular processes are very fast: agents don't have to think about, or wait for their perceptions to come online. Speed and mandatoriness go hand in hand (Fodor 1983, 63–64);

(5) *Informational encapsulation:* The input from modules is encapsulated, which is to say that "cognitive modules have no access to information from elsewhere in the cognitive system (except of course for the initial input into an output system)" (Guttenplan 1995, 443). Fodor cites visual illusions, such as the perception that two equidistant lines are unequal in length in the Müller-Lyer illusion, to demonstrate information encapsulation. Even when an agent knows that the two lines are of equal length, it is nonetheless the case that his visual perception may lead him to think that one line is longer than the other (Fodor 1983, 66);

(6) *Shallow output:* Fodor makes use of a contrast between *observation* (what modules do) and *inferences* about the content of those observations. Modules observe, but do not make inferences;

(7) *Fixed neural architecture:* Modular activities are localized into certain parts of the brain, a claim that marries nicely with the claim that modular activities are domain specific;

(8) *Characteristic and specific breakdown pattern:* This property can be understood as a consequence of the previous property: if each module is localized, then it is possible for one to break down, in isolation, while the other modules remain intact;

(9) *Ontogenetic systems which exhibit characteristic pace and sequencing:* Empirical research seems to bear out that mental subsystems such as perception and language ability share this characteristic.

Philip Gerrans points out that one of the drawbacks of modularity theses is that "A mind composed entirely of such perceptual and quasi-perceptual input and output modules would be quite rigid, stimulus bound, and unable to cope with novel situations with exceed its online first-order representational capacities" (Gerrans 2002, 305).

Humans, however, have more mental flexibility, and are not hamstrung by modularity. Even if the mind is modular in some respects, no modularity theorist believes that all capacities of the mind are modular. According to Fodor, modular cognitive systems are innately specified, as opposed to being formed by "some sort of learning process" (Fodor 1983, 37). But there is surely room for those activities of the mind that are informed by a learning process, such as the scientific method, or art history, activities that are dependent upon central processes as opposed to modular ones.

With this understanding of modularity, the question remains as to whether theory of mind is modular in nature, and if so, what difference this might make. Baron-Cohen suggests that a modular subsystem may account for theory of mind (Baron-Cohen 1995, 57). Brian J. Scholl and Alan M. Leslie (1999) argue that theory of mind is an excellent candidate for a modular process, as the metarepresentational aspects of theory of mind are not likely to be empirically acquired. Rather, "the capacity to acquire [theory of mind] has a specific innate basis" (Scholl and Leslie 1999, 133). On the other side of the debate are those who believe that theory of mind may be accounted for via other processes, such as simulations, or a generalized mechanism for theory acquisition and building.

The fact that theory of mind appears to be domain-specific, encapsulated, and that it may arise from an innate part of human cognitive architecture, supports the thesis that theory of mind is modular in nature. If autism simply is a condition in which theory of mind is selectively impaired, then the modularity thesis is strengthened. Scholl and Leslie argue against those who would discount theory of mind as a modular process because of its ability to develop, as well as theory of mind's ability to be affected by environmental factors. It is uncontroversial that theory of mind develops over the course of a typical child's early life—theory of mind is not mature before the age of three, but by the age of four, most children are far more adept at the false-belief tasks that indicate facility with theory of mind. But this developing capacity should not disqualify theory of mind from modularity, as there is nothing in the modularity thesis that precludes the possibility of development. The likelihood that modules would "'come online,' often through intermediate states" is entirely consistent with canonical modular accounts (Scholl and Leslie 1999, 136). Even mature modules can develop.[17]

Environment can have an affect on the development of theory of mind, but Scholl and Leslie argue that this does not undermine the modularity of theory of mind. Children with siblings typically demonstrate facility with theory of mind earlier than children without siblings, but the significant lesson is that there is *uniformity of outcome in theory of mind,* even if the developmental path is shorter or longer due to environmental influences. "Children with many siblings don't develop *different* [theories of mind]; they just do it a bit earlier" (Scholl and Leslie 1999, 139). Garfield et al. hold that theory of mind is modular, although it is "neither encapsulated nor innately determined" (Garfield et al. 2001, 534). Part of the complexity in determining whether a theory of mind module exists is that there is no uniform agreement about the appropriate characteristics of modules.

Gerrans argues that the evidence from autism does not demonstrate that a theory of mind module exists. Instead, he holds that "the alleged modularity of [theory of mind] results from interpreting the outcome of developmental failures characteristic of autism at too high a level of cognitive abstraction" (Gerrans 2002, 305). Gerrans does not dispute the existence of mental modules. Rather, autism is the result of a failure of a module other than a theory of mind module: autism is "not a result of damage to a mindreading module but the result of neurological damage to a number of early cognitive mechanisms whose proper function is essential to the development of mindreading" (Gerrans 2002, 314). Evidence for this claim includes the facts that mindreading difficulties are not the sole deficit facing persons with autism, and that some of those deficits cannot be accounted for by a lack of theory of mind alone. Garfield et al. concur with Gerrans, holding that empirical evidence supports "the innateness of the *processes and structures subserving* [theory of mind], coupled with the relative uniformity of the relevant social and environmental parameters, and not the innateness of [theory of mind], *per se* . . ." (Garfield et al. 2002, 499). Some of the additional problems faced by persons with autism which Gerrans cites to support his hypothesis include sensorimotor problems, echolalia, or unusual physical sensitivities. Here Gerrans anticipates Shanker's (2004) hypothesis, discussed earlier. Nor, in Gerrans's estimation, do theory of mind deficits adequately account for some of the strengths evidenced by some persons with autism, such as superior memory or other islets of intelligence (Gerrans 2002, 315–316). Gerrans concludes that it would make more sense to look for a deeper cause, rather than a failure of a single theory of mind module. Rather than embrace a weak central coherence or weak executive function account, Gerrans argues that a deficit in a social processing module would have more explanatory strength than an explanation based on a theory of mind module.[18] Gerrans does not argue that persons with autism succeed in having functioning theories of mind; rather, their theory of mind failures are due to the cognitive prerequisites for mindreading, which are more plausible candidates for modules (Gerrans 2002, 318). Thus, Gerrans concludes that there is no theory of mind module.

Alison Gopnik et al. concur in part with Gerrans, holding that while there is an innate basis for the theory of mind, a modularity thesis of theory of mind is incorrect (Gopnik et al. 2000). Rather than saying that theory of mind per se is innate, they cite evidence for the claim that successive theories of mind are formed, revised, and replaced. Thus, *theory formulation* is innate, and not any one particular theory of mind. Garfield et al. (2001) reject Gopnik et al.'s position, as it requires too much sophistication about theories at too young an age. On this view, persons with autism have a general weakness in theory formation, which also accounts for their difficulties in employing TT and ST. Gopnik et al.'s position marries well with the weak central coherence theory of autism—if a person has difficulty with theory development and execution in general, it would stand to reason that he would be more interested in surfaces and details, rather than coherent wholes (Gopnik et al. 2000, 66).

If the executive function theory or central coherence theory are true, this does not necessarily demonstrate anything about the modularity of theory of mind. Perhaps weak executive function or weak central coherence prevents individuals from accessing their theory of mind modules; thus there may be a theory of mind module that is nonetheless inoperative in cases of autism. On the other hand, weak executive function or weak central coherence might cause an individual to have a weakened theory of mind, if executive function or central coherence are causal precursors to theory of mind. Such a theory calls into question the possibility that a dedicated theory of mind module exists (Glüer and Pagin 2003). The evidence from autism is not conclusive.

Gerrans may be mistaken on two counts. First, theory of mind deficits may account for more than previously assumed. For example, the hypothesis that persons with autism excel at folk physics to the same extent that they perform poorly on folk psychological tasks is a parsimonious means by which the theory of mind account explains not merely social and communication deficits, but also ritualized or obsessive behaviors. Second, even if theory of mind deficits do not account for every aspect of autism, that fact is not sufficient to conclude that there is no theory of mind module at all. Less ambitious conclusions, such as the claim that autism is accounted for by damage both to a theory of mind module and to some other mental subsystem, may serve just as well. As stated above, the weak central coherence and weak executive function thesis do not preclude the theory of mind thesis.

A final position in the modularity debate is staked out by Max Coltheart and Robyn Langdon. They do not deny that mental modules may exist, but rather hold that the evidence from autism points to the claim that "autism is not a single homogeneous condition, and so can have no single cause" (Coltheart and Langdon 1998, 138). The assumption that all persons with autism have the same cognitive abnormality, as well as the assumption that all of the symptoms of autism are caused by that single abnormality, are false (Coltheart and Langdon 1998, 139). Rather, autism should be understood as a "multidimensional spectrum of symptoms that co-occur independently" (Coltheart and Langdon 1998, 139). They draw analogies between autism and other cognitive disorders, such as Broca's aphasia or schizophrenia—conditions in which not every symptom associated with the disorder co-occurs in every case. Furthermore, functional modularity and anatomical modularity do not necessarily go hand in hand: individuals can have different areas of the brain damaged, and yet evidence identical symptoms as a result of very different forms of brain damage. Thus, the claim that modules have a fixed neural architecture is questioned. The wide diversity of symptoms exhibited by persons with autism, and the varying degrees to which different individuals with autism can have different symptoms, bolster their conclusions. Coltheart and Langdon state that the lessons are both to "eschew syndromes"—why believe that the lowest functioning person with autism and the highest-functioning person with Asperger's have the same disorder?—and eschew localization. Rather than make the *syndrome* the object of study, since there may not be a unitary syndrome, Coltheart and Langdon urge that the *symptom* must be the subject of the study. They do not abandon the modularity thesis, only caution that "the development of an adequately fine-grained abstract theory of the structure of cognitive systems must precede any attempts to map the neural substrate of cognition" (Coltheart and Langdon 1998, 151).

Three significant lessons emerge from the modularity debate. First, it is clear that there is much that is still unknown about autism and the mind in general. Psychologists and philosophers are further along than Leontius in his travels outside the city walls, but there is much distance yet to be covered. Second, assumptions about uniformity across cases of autism are probably mistaken. Coltheart and Langdon are right to conclude that the focus should be the *symptoms*, and not the *syndrome*. In keeping with this important point, this book focuses primarily on the implications of the lack of theory of mind, and persons with autism who lack theory of mind.

Not every person with autism lacks theory of mind, and not every person who lacks theory of mind has autism. Some high-functioning persons with autism, including those with Asperger's syndrome, do have a theory of mind.[19] As stated earlier, between 20 and 35 percent of persons with autism pass false-belief tasks, although the number decreases significantly when persons with autism are challenged with second-order, rather than first-order, false-belief tasks. Another population with deficits in reciprocal understanding consistent with a lack of theory of mind is psychopaths. Psychopathy is characterized by "a profound affective bluntness towards the past, the future, and anything human. . . . [T]he psychopath's portrait consistently emerged as depicting a manipulative, grandiose, and superficial parasite, who, devoid of emotional connections to the world, irresponsibly and selfishly drifts though life, only stopping long enough to callously, impulsively, and aggressively satisfy the urge of the moment" (Hervé 2007, 45). While there are some who hold that psychopaths may be characterized by executive function deficits (Herba et al. 2007, 260), there are significant differences between persons with autism and psychopaths. Frith distinguishes between the two populations in the following way: while both groups demonstrate a lack of empathy in some cases, psychopaths are tremendously good at mentalizing. Additionally, while persons with autism are able to make distinctions between moral and conventional rules,[20] psychopaths are not able to do so (Frith 2003, 114). Jeannette Kennett claims that the distinction lies in the autistic person's ability to recognize the interests of others as reason-giving, and the psychopath's indifference to those interests:

> Autistic people, though lacking empathy, do seem capable of deep moral concerns. They are capable, as psychopaths are not, of the subjective realization that other people's interests are reason-giving in the same way as one's own, though they may have great difficulty in discerning what those interests are. It is not the psychopath's lack of empathy, which (on its own, at any rate) explains his moral indifference. It is more specifically his lack of concern, or more likely the lack of capacity to understand what he is doing, to consider the reasons available to him and to act in accordance with them. (Kennett 2002, 354)

This does not undermine the earlier claims about the autistic person's inability to employ TT or ST. An individual can recognize that certain facts are reason-giving, although not have the means by which to know what those facts are. Once John clearly presented Marci with the facts that he was cold and that he thought that closing the window would relieve the draft, Marci would understand why he closed the window, even if she was unable to use TT or ST to figure this out in lieu of the explicit presentation of John's intentions. The psychopath has the means—theory of mind—by which he might determine reasons for treating people in a certain way, but he is indifferent to those reasons.

If Marci was psychopathic, even if she was well aware of John's discomfort, and well aware of her close proximity to the window, Marci would not see these facts as a reason to do anything at all. Kennett may not be on firm ground drawing a distinction between the autistic person and the psychopath by claiming that the psychopath "lacks capacity to understand what he is doing," given Frith and Happé's discussion of the lack of introspection on the part of persons with autism. However, Kennett's point about the psychopath's indifference to reason-giving attitudes on the part of others is uncontested.

Even with these exceptions, however, theory of mind and theory of mind deficits remain one of the best descriptions of the complex combination of symptoms that affect persons with autism. The third lesson of the modularity debate follows from the first two: what it might mean to "cure" someone with autism is much more complex than could possibly be understood today. So much about the mind is yet to be understood. So much about autism is yet to be understood. Ethics will not herald the end of autism. That much is known. But understanding the ethics of autism is invaluable in knowing how to best answer moral questions that emerge among the autistic and non-autistic communities. Who is the autistic person, and what do we owe him? A better understanding of that question, and the complexity of its answer, is found in the next chapter.

Voices of Autism

Wendy Lawson recounts her first forty-two years in her autobiography, Life Behind Glass. During most of her life Lawson was wrongly diagnosed with schizophrenia. She endured the death of her infant brother, the near-amputation of one of her legs along with attendant operations and physical therapy, difficulties in school, her parents' divorce, two brief institutionalizations, and her own divorce before she was diagnosed with Asperger's syndrome as an adult. Despite these setbacks, Lawson's life is also marked by personal triumphs: a brief but fulfilling career in nursing, raising four children, successful emigration to Australia, and the completion of several college degrees.

Autism created a variety of obstacles in Lawson's life. She was plagued by sensory sensitivities in her childhood, although less so in adulthood. The mysteries of human relationships are a pervasive theme in her writing. She cautions those who would make friends with someone who is autistic that "the autistic person needs to manipulate their surroundings in other to maintain a sense of control of their environment"; this manipulation can extend to those with whom autistic people try to relate (Lawson 1998, 19). Reciprocal relationships can come, but they are hard-won. Lawson made friends in her life, and was married. Her first close friend was a woman named Lesley whom Lawson praises as someone who recognized Lawson as valuable on her own terms (Lawson 1998, 49). But many friendships, as well as her marriage, were transient. Looking back, Lawson says after only after two decades of marriage and four years of divorce was she "beginning to understand what an adult communicative relationship actually means" (Lawson 1998, 68).

Lawson recognizes that her interactions with people are quite different from others she observes, including those in television or in books (Lawson 1998, 8). She attributes some of her difficulties in connecting with others to behaviors that might appear "bizarre or embarrassing" (Lawson 1998, 110). Near the end of her autobiography she acknowledges that her relationships with others may be compromised by the fact that "I still find it very difficult to put myself 'in the other person's shoes.' I can only feel my needs and myself—everything outside is foreign and alien to me" (Lawson 1998, 113).

In personal communication with Wendy in 2007, she added these thoughts to her insights in Life Behind Glass:

> In my book, Life Behind Glass, I describe the experience of feeling 'connected' to another person: "The sun was warm on our bodies and the dappled shade of nearby trees flickered across our faces as we laughed together. It was good to laugh and to feel accepted in the company of another." These days I experience much acceptance and love by both family and friends. Being valued enough to have my particular learning style accommodated is vital to my current appreciation of life. At the same time I am able to share my experiences with others and shed light on much of my autistic world. This is my passion. I love teaching and helping others to 'see' something that, perhaps, they had been blind to before. Words are a tool I use to build connections to experiences, understanding and everyday 'normality.' I hope they might become stepping stones to a more inclusive society and be useful in promoting a better future for the autistic children of our day.

2

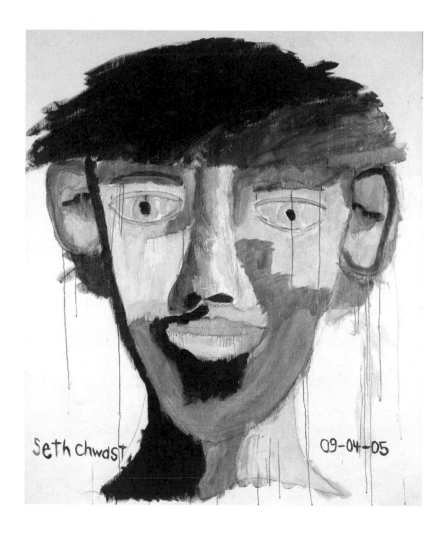

SETH CHWAST, *SELF-STUDY IN BLUE GREEN*

The Value of an Autistic Life

Much philosophical energy has been expended on questions such as: What makes an individual a "person"? What makes a human life a "good human life," a life that has gone well? What makes an individual a "member of the moral community"? The differences between each of these distinctions help to map out moral obligations. "Human" is a biological sorting concept. A "good human life" is one that would be fulfilling, or one that would allow a human to flourish, given the kind of biological entity that a human is. "Persons" are those individuals who should be given a certain moral standing, such as moral rights; the set of "persons" may not be co-extensive with the set of "humans." In claiming that the two sets are not co-extensive one may claim that some non-humans deserve special moral consideration, or that some biological humans are not worthy of the same moral consideration as other humans. "Members of the moral community" are those persons with whom other persons share moral obligations. The difficult question lies not in determining the intension of each of these terms, but in mapping out the extensions: what is the set of individuals captured by each of these terms?

Some people bristle at these questions. Attempts to answer these questions can be a prelude to exclusion, discrimination, or oppression. Martha Nussbaum cites three objections to this type of project. First, dominant groups have historically defined the "human" in their own image, thereby further marginalizing the oppressed. Second, narrow definitions may restrict individuals from autonomously carrying out their own plans for life. For example, if it is concluded that certain groups do not really need an education to pursue a life worth living, then the conclusion that it is morally acceptable to withhold education can follow. Finally, even when the conception of the "human" is drawn as fairly as possible, the powerless can still be excluded (Nussbaum 1995). Nussbaum is not persuaded to suspend her inquiry into human nature by any of these objections, although she recognizes the historical injustices that have resulted from such a project. Eva Feder Kittay believes that those who would claim that "such intrinsic psychological capacities as rationality and autonomy are requisites for claims of justice, a good quality of life, and the moral considerations of personhood" are making arguments that are as morally repugnant as arguments that argue for exclusion on the basis of physical disability or race (Kittay 2005, 100). Thin analyses of these questions that attempt to draw distinctions based upon a single factor—IQ, for example— are bound to be both philosophically weak and prone to Nussbaum's objections.[1]

While this type of inquiry can result in harms to the oppressed or powerless, it can also be a prelude to actions that are designed to improve people's lives: how can we undertake the actions needed to improve human lives unless we have some sense of what makes for a good human life? Robert M. Veatch (1999), for example, recognizes the relevance of posing questions about the nature of a good human life to surrogate decision making for patients who are temporarily incompetent. In the absence of informed consent from a patient or a surrogate, physicians may be forced to make medical decisions based on what would be in a patient's best interest; but without a conception of what it means for a life to go well, physicians are unable to make a judgment about what course of action would be in a patient's best interest. Thus, answers to these questions can be both of tremendous value and the basis of discrimination and oppression. The questions are not damaging; what is damaging is what we do with the answers.

What follows is not an exhaustive account of philosophers' answers to these questions. An exhaustive account would be a book—at least—in its own right. Rather, what follows is a sampling of attempts to answer these questions. Some of these accounts have significant overlap, while others have less in common. The goal is to establish common threads among philosophical accounts, and see what can be woven from those common threads. No argument is offered in favor of one account over the others, although objections are offered to the last account presented. The objective here is not to determine which of these accounts is correct. Rather, the discussion focuses on those common threads, and what those common threads hold for persons with autism who lack a theory of mind.

The discussion is not meant to be exhaustive in scope, but to present a variety of perspectives with an eye toward common overlap. The positions were initially presented in the context of both moral theory (Scanlon, Nussbaum, and Parfit), and bioethics (Warren and Veatch). Only two positions (Hobson and Benn) were crafted with the autistic person in mind, although Nussbaum considers the implications of her position for a person with Asperger's (Nussbaum 2006). All of the discussants are contemporary philosophers, but it is clear that some of their views are informed by historical perspectives. Warren, Hobson, and Benn focus on one question: what makes a human a person, such that he has moral rights, or deserves moral consideration from others? Nussbaum, Scanlon, Veatch, and Parfit focus on a second question: what makes a human life a good life?

Ultimately, answers to these questions will help us answer questions about the moral obligations shared between the autistic and non-autistic community. The discussion in chapter 3 concerns theories that best determine the moral status of actions among autistic and non-autistic persons. The need for such theories assumes that persons with autism are members of the moral community; thus, the conclusions reached here will have significant repercussions. The discussion in chapter 4 of the use of genetic technologies and autism is predicated on whether an autistic life is in fact a well-lived human life. Finally, the discussion in chapter 5 of the use of adults with autism in some types of biomedical research turns on these same questions about a well-lived human life.

Unquestionably, a great deal is at stake here.

Warren on Membership in the Moral Community

Mary Anne Warren considers a set of conditions that are "most central to the concept of personhood, or humanity in the moral sense" (Warren 1996, 67). Warren presents these criteria toward establishing the moral permissibility of abortion: if it can be established that a fetus is not a person, that is, a fetus does not have a moral right not to be killed equal to a woman's moral right to perform an abortion, then it can be shown that abortions can be morally permissible. Warren believes that questions of abortion are not answered by an examination of the fetus's status as a human, but instead on the basis of personhood, or membership in the moral community: "A fetus cannot be considered a member of the moral community, the set of beings with full and equal moral rights, for the simple reason that it is not a person, and [that] it is personhood, and not genetic humanity, i.e., humanity defined by Noonan, which is the basis for membership in this community" (Warren 1996, 62).[2]

It is possible to object to Warren's claim that personhood, and not humanness, determines the permissibility of some abortions, or to object to her project in defending abortion on other grounds. This is, however, not the object of the present inquiry. Instead, the object is to see what Warren says about personhood and membership in the moral community, and to see if any interesting lessons can be drawn from her claims. In arguing for the premise that fetuses are not persons, that is, not members of the moral community with a full right to life, Warren delineates what properties an individual must have in order to have moral personhood. Warren presents the following five criteria (Warren 1996, 67):

(1) consciousness (of objects and events external and/or internal to the being), and in particular the capacity to feel pain;

(2) reasoning (the *developed* capacity to solve new and relative complex problems);

(3) self-motivated activity (activity which is relatively independent of either genetic or direct external control);

(4) the capacity to communicate, by whatever means, messages of an indefinite variety of types, that is, not just with an

indefinite number of possible contents, but on indefinitely many possible topics;

(5) the presence of self-concepts, and self-awareness, either individual or racial, or both.

Warren does not present an argument for each of these criteria, but rather, a thought-experiment: if humans were to discover aliens, what would be the basis for claiming that these aliens were worthy of moral consideration and not merely, as Warren puts it, "a source of food"? Were we to learn that the non-human aliens had many of the above properties, we would regard them as having moral standing. Warren does not claim that all five of the above are jointly necessary or sufficient for moral personhood; she claims that perhaps only (1) and (2) are jointly sufficient for moral personhood and that "quite probably (1)–(3) are sufficient" (Warren 1996, 67). Warren also claims that criteria (1) and (2) are candidates for necessary conditions for personhood, and as long as (3) is construed to include "the activity of reasoning," then (3) may also be a necessary condition for personhood.

While criteria (2) and (3) are interesting, the most intriguing questions arise with respect to Warren's first criterion. What precisely does Warren mean by the consciousness of objects and events both *internal* and *external* to the being whose consciousness is under consideration? In chapter 1 the question was raised as to whether the consciousness of persons with autism might be fundamentally different from the consciousness of non-autistic persons. It is taken for granted in most cases that if an agent *believes that P*, then the agent *believes that he believes P*. Introspection of one's conscious states is part of what it is to be conscious of those internal states. The possibility that persons with autism are conscious, but not conscious of their intentional states, was raised. If an agent's self-awareness is a cognitive achievement, to use Raffman's terminology introduced in chapter 1, then this would account for why it was that persons lacking theory of mind would be unable to introspect their own conscious states. Warren claims that members of the moral community must have consciousness of *events internal to themselves*. Does this necessitate that members of the moral community are able to introspect their conscious states, or is it enough that they are conscious, without consciousness of that consciousness?

One response to this concern is to draw a distinction between consciousness and self-consciousness, claiming that while consciousness is either necessary or sufficient for personhood, self-consciousness is a separate property which is neither necessary nor sufficient for personhood. Warren's fifth criterion concerns self-consciousness, implying that self-consciousness is distinct from consciousness. In Warren's estimation, self-consciousness is not as significant in determining moral personhood as consciousness itself. Perhaps a lack of introspection on the part of the person with autism alleged by Frith and Happé is not so problematic using Warren's criteria of personhood.

Before concerns about an agent's internal conscious states can be put to rest, however, Warren's claims about the capacity to feel pain merit examination. As noted in chapter 1, Raffman claims that agents are in a privileged position with respect to their conscious occurrent sensations. Pain is certainly a candidate for a conscious occurrent sensation. Does Warren's first criterion assert that the individual in question must be *aware of pain when they are in pain,* or is *being in pain* enough? Perhaps members of the moral community do not need to have self-consciousness in order to have consciousness, but they may need to have awareness of pain to be in pain. In most cases, awareness of pain is both necessary and sufficient for being in pain. If you are aware of pain, then you are in pain; similarly, if an agent is not aware of pain, then that agent is not in pain. This straightforward position, which would take the first-person reports of persons with autism at face value, would be embraced by McGeer. One of the results of a failure of introspection on the part of persons with autism, however, is that they may be unaware even of occurrent sensations such as pain. Thus, the claim that awareness of pain is necessary for being in pain may not hold for the autistic individual.[3] Frith and Happé cite in their discussion an example of "a young girl with autism who was found to have suffered acute appendicitis, but had not complained of any pain and, when asked how she felt, did not report anything wrong" (Frith and Happé 1999, 10). This is only one example; to draw broad generalizations on the basis of one girl's experiences would be ill-advised. But the girl's experiences, coupled with Frith and Happé's intriguing work on the consciousness of persons with autism, do raise important questions.

In addition to the questions that are raised with respect to consciousness of *internal* objects and events, consciousness of *external* objects and events should also be investigated. Understanding Warren's claim that members of the moral community are conscious of *objects and events external* to that being requires a more complete understanding of the notion of consciousness. "Consciousness" is an intrinsic property, a property that a being has in and of itself. "Consciousness" is not a property that a thing has or loses because of the way that something else in the world happens to be. Some properties are best understood as relations, rather than as intrinsic properties—the property itself depends on a relationship between the thing that has the property and some other thing. "Prey" is a property that something has only if it stands in a special relationship to something else: unless there is something out there that is hunting *A*, it does not make much sense to say of *A* that it is prey. "Consciousness" is not a relation, but "prey" certainly is. *No one doubts that persons with autism are conscious of other persons.* But the question is, are individuals with autism conscious of other persons *qua* persons? Warren's first criterion does not address this question. Consciousness, on the face of it, does not necessitate that members of the moral community have relationships, or even the capacity for relationships, with other moral persons. Must members of the moral community merely be conscious of the fact that something else is there, or must they respond in a way that demonstrates their consciousness is a consciousness of a particular *kind* of thing? If consciousness is directed toward an object of some kind, then consciousness of other persons *qua* persons implies taking the intentional stance toward those who are intentional agents. An inability to take the intentional stance could call into question an individual's claim to consciousness in a robust sense.

A vivid example of this type of interaction is recounted by Katharine P. Beals, describing interactions with her autistic son Jason:

> We were constantly losing him, constantly chasing after him to try to reengage him, constantly reminded, in his failure to respond, of all that escaped him. "Wow, Jason, look at how fast you've got that plate spinning," I'd say to him as he scurried off to admire it from a distance, my voice breaking, and tears escaping, as I thought of how

far he was from ever being able to understand what I'd said, or even that I was a person with thoughts and feelings, not a wind-up toy. I'd tickle him, and he'd look at my hands; I'd chase him, and he'd watch my feet; I'd put a flashlight in my mouth, and he'd stare at the flashlight. (Beals 2003, 36)

Jason does not walk into his mother as if she did not exist, or treat her as if she were invisible. But since he does not take the intentional stance toward her, did he genuinely have consciousness of her *qua* person? The failure to take the intentional stance is a particularly egregious mistake, different from other mistakes about persons. For example, it is possible to take the intentional stance toward another person in the room, but fail to recognize that the other person is a stranger who did not know on which shelf the juice is kept. In such a case there would be consciousness of another person, in the relevant ways, even though there was not conscious of some facts about that person. A person does not have to be conscious of *everything* about another person to enter into a relationship with that person. But a person does need to be conscious of the fact that this other individual is in fact a person with beliefs, intentions, wants and desires. Without that consciousness, an essential part of the relationship would be compromised.

Of course, it is possible that the consciousness that Warren is speaking of is not consciousness of anything *qua* the kind of thing that it is. As long as Jason is conscious of something in his way—a human form, a flashlight—that is enough. But for those who believe that part of consciousness is getting it right, Jason's mistake—so heartbreaking because it is so crucial—raises significant questions.

In summary, Warren sets out a criterion—consciousness—without elaborating on what consciousness might consist in. This raises a question: can the person lacking theory of mind be said to be conscious of other persons *qua* persons, given his lack of theory of mind? Some might argue that all that is essential for consciousness of other persons is an awareness that something is there, even if the individual who had awareness of the other person was entirely wrong about the nature of persons. Rather than attempting to explain other persons using TT, ST, or any other strategy available to the folk psychologist, a person with autism might consider other persons to be elaborate puzzles in folk physics. Perhaps this thin awareness of other persons is enough to qualify for "consciousness." Others may take a stronger stance: if you are not conscious of persons *qua* persons, in what sense are you conscious of a person at all?

Nussbaum on Human Capabilities

Martha Nussbaum's discussion of human capabilities is presented both as part of a feminist response to relativistic thinking that harms women (Nussbaum 1995) and an attempt to improve upon social contract theories that come up short when considering questions about the disabled, global justice, and animal rights (Nussbaum 2006). Nussbaum challenges versions of moral relativism that claim that cultural difference makes it morally permissible for some women to have fewer opportunities than men, or for women to endure institutionalized illiteracy, or suffer inadequate nutrition (Nussbaum 1995). Cultural differences cannot be cited as a justification for such practices, Nussbaum claims, because such practices fail to take into consideration universal capabilities shared among humans, and universal conceptions of a good human life that follow from these shared capabilities. Women and men are human, they share the same capabilities, and in virtue of these shared capabilities, they share what it is for their lives to go well or poorly. The first step in her argument against cultural relativism that leads to oppression is to ask "What are the characteristic activities of the human being? What does the human being do, characteristically, as such—and not, say as a member of a particular group, or a particular local community?" (Nussbaum 1995, 72). Nussbaum recognizes that her project is essentialist—she is making claims about properties she considers universal to human beings. Usurpation of these capabilities does harm to any human.

Nussbaum observes that the result of her project is not merely descriptive, but also prescriptive. Without these capabilities, a human being would be unable to flourish, and in fact "we can argue, by imagining a life without the capability in quest, that such a life is not a life worthy of human dignity" (Nussbaum 2006, 78). While "human" is typically understood to be a biological designation, Nussbaum's project is not about biology per se, but rather is an ethical inquiry. She observes that some philosophers who have undertaken this project do so in an attempt to understand what it means to be a person, although she eschews this term because it has legal precedents that entail masculinity, and she is looking for a gender-neutral understanding of human capabilities (Nussbaum 1995). What follows is a summary of Nussbaum's list of the central human capabilities (Nussbaum 2006):[4]

(1) *life:* humans have a normal lifespan which they should be permitted to live out with a life worth living;

(2) *bodily health:* humans should be able to have good health, have adequate nourishment and shelter;

(3) *bodily integrity:* humans should have the ability to move freely from place to place, be secure against violent assault, and opportunities for sexual satisfaction and choice in reproduction;

(4) *senses, imagination, and thought:* humans have the freedom to use their senses, as well as to think, imagine, and reason in a "truly human way" about a variety of issues, and the freedom to express themselves;

(5) *emotions:* "being able to have attachments to things and people outside ourselves; to love those who love and care for us, to grieve at their absence; in general to love, to grieve, to experience longing, gratitude, and justified anger" (Nussbaum 2006, 76–77);

(6) *practical reason:* humans are able to form a conception of the good and participate (or try to) in planning and managing their own lives;

(7) *affiliation with other human beings:* humans recognize and feel some sense of affiliation with other human beings; this is also the social basis of self-respect and nonhumiliation;

(8) humans experience a *relatedness to other species and to nature;*

(9) humans experience *humor and play;*

(10) *control over one's environment:* freedom of political choice, as well as material choice of property rights and employment.

Nussbaum takes this list as a jumping-off point for answering further questions: what is the threshold at which a life is so impoverished that it fails to be a human life, and what is the threshold at which a life is a human life, but not a good human life (Nussbaum 1995)? Nussbaum spends little time on the first question, although her discussion does touch upon the status of persons in persistent vegetative states, persons with severe dementia, and severely damaged infants. While this list does tell us what we owe to those who are human, this does not tell us what we morally owe to those individuals who fall short on her list. With respect to the second question, however, she notes that "a life that lacks any one of these capacities, no matter what else it has, will fall short of being a good human life" (Nussbaum 1995). Elsewhere she notes that without a number of these capabilities, "such a life is not a life worthy of human dignity" (Nussbaum 2006, 78), or at the very least is not a life of human "flourishing" (Nussbaum 2006, 86). It is not enough to lack for any one of these capabilities, but if several are missing, that can be sufficient for a life to either fail to be a human life, or to be a human life that is not worth living (Nussbaum 2006, 181).

The fifth and seventh criteria are of importance to a discussion of the autistic individual. Nussbaum states that the universal experience of infantile dependency "gives rise to a great deal of overlapping experience that is central in the formation of desires, and of complex emotions such as grief, love, and anger. This, in turn, is a major source of our ability to recognize ourselves in the emotional experiences of those whose lives are very different in other respects from our own" (Nussbaum 1995, 78). The recognition of others' emotional experiences is important to human life. When considering the importance of affiliation with other human beings, there is an implicit recognition that it is not mere affiliation with something, but *something in particular* that is an essential human capability. One of the challenges facing persons with autism with an impoverished theory of mind is the inability to recognize others' emotional experiences.[5] Uta Frith discusses the difficulties faced by the autistic person who lacks a theory of mind, who is unable to "mentalize," or take an intentional stance toward others:

Intentional empathy, however, does require an ability to mentalize, and is thus dependent on the instinctive orientation to other people's mental states. This is the way in which Baron-Cohen uses the term "empathizing" when characterizing social impairments in autism. This type of empathy is linked to understanding the reasons for another person's sadness or fear, and with the appropriate response. The appropriate response depends on the situation and this is precisely where a theory of mind comes into its own. This is not an occasion for fixed rules. In one case, the appropriate empathetic response may be turning away and leaving the distressed person alone; in another case, it may be giving comfort by word or deed; and in yet another situation the appropriate response may be to join with outrage. (Frith 2003, 112)

The parallels between Frith's observations and Nussbaum's are telling:

Thus, when other people suffer capability failure, the citizen I imagine will not simply feel the sentiments required by moral impartiality, viewed as a constraint on her own pursuit of self-interest. Instead, she will feel compassion for them *as a part of her own good.* (Nussbaum 2006, 91)

The connection between Frith and Nussbaum is clear: not only will the person who lacks this empathetic ability live a life that is not a good human life, a life whose good is compromised in virtue of being unable to make certain empathetic connections, but that individual may also lack the capacity to perform the morally right action in certain situations. The points made here marry well with those made in Nussbaum's seventh criterion. With limited empathy, ability to mentalize, or theory of mind, can the person with autism possess the sense of affiliation that Nussbaum requires? As observed by McGeer in chapter 1, this is a problem not only for the person with autism, but it is a problem for the non-autistic person also. Without a shared experience of empathy, neither group can understand the other. The gulf between the two is substantial.

Nussbaum elaborates on the sixth capacity by saying that individuals who "altogether lack" the ability to choose and evaluate their life plans, including "what is good and how one should live . . . would not be likely to be regarded as fully human, in any society" (Nussbaum 1995, 78). A departure between Warren and Nussbaum is apparent.

Warren makes the following claim: if S does not have the property of moral personhood, then S does not have full moral rights. This is the basis for her claim that a fetus, which is nonetheless a biological human and is killed by abortion, may permissibly be killed in certain circumstances. Individuals who fail to meet Warren's criteria for personhood are not members of the moral community, and as such, they do not have full moral rights. Members of the moral community do not have the same obligations to those individuals who fail to meet the criteria of personhood as they do toward those who are members of the moral community. Does Nussbaum agree? Her discussion of the sixth criterion touches on the connection between agency, volition, and moral obligation. Nussbaum states that those unable to act in keeping with practical reason—who lack agency in this sense—are "not likely to be regarded as fully human." But Nussbaum also states explicitly that the failure of an individual to be "fully human" does not demonstrate anything about what is owed to that individual. Thus, Nussbaum denies the strong claim that Warren makes between the moral personhood of an individual and the obligations that others have to that individual. For Nussbaum, it is possible not to be regarded as fully human, and yet still be an individual to whom we owe moral obligations. Warren's position is stronger and more exclusivist than Nussbaum's.

Another aspect of Nussbaum's sixth criterion is the claim that part of practical reason is the ability to make choices in keeping with what is good—not merely good to the individual, but good *simpliciter*. Practical reason is not merely about choosing what we want, or what fulfills our own desires, it is also about choosing what is good. Nussbaum is suggesting that there is an objective fact about what is good. What might that be? Thomas Scanlon attempts to answer this question.

Scanlon, Veatch, and Parfit on the Elements of Well-Being

Derek Parfit presents a detailed and influential discussion of personhood, focusing primarily on questions about personal identity over time (Parfit 1984). Thomas Scanlon does not directly address questions about what makes a person a person, but instead considers what makes a person's life a good life, the second of Nussbaum's questions. Scanlon considers three different types of theories that answer questions about what makes a person's life go well, significantly informed by Derek Parfit (Scanlon 1998; Parfit 1984). The first are what Scanlon refers to as "experiential theories," which hold that the experiences that one has, or seems to have, determine the goodness of a person's life. Scanlon dismisses experiential theories as misguided because according to such an account an agent's life would be just as good when filled with false, but seemingly loyal friends, as a life filled with steadfast friends. Intuitively, a life filled with seemingly loyal but false friends would not be as good as one that was filled with true friends, even if the agent in question never knew the difference. The second are what Scanlon calls "desire theories" which claim that the degree to which a person's desires are fulfilled determines the goodness of that person's life. Scanlon does not dismiss this account as quickly as the experiential account, but he ultimately does reject it. For one, it would seem that a person could have desires that have nothing whatsoever to do with her well-being, or which actively thwart her well-being, such as the desire to smoke. To have these desires fulfilled would not contribute in any way to the goodness of her life. Second, on this account a person could arbitrarily add to her list of desires ("I desire that there are eggs at the grocery store," "I desire that tomorrow be Tuesday") and once fulfilled, have her well-being increase. This seems absurd. Attempts to circumvent these problems often lead to an "informed desire" theory. But even if a person has "informed desires," there remains a question. Why is the fulfillment of certain desires, or certain types of desires, more conducive to well-being than others? Scanlon believes that this question can be answered by introducing rational aims—a good life becomes one in which that which is worthwhile and valuable is pursued. Once the notion of objective claims about that which is worthwhile and good are introduced, the desire theory evolves into a third type of theory, which Scanlon refers to as "substantive good" or "objective list" theories. According to these theories, there are "standards for assessing the quality of a life that are not entirely dependent on the desires of the person whose life it is" (Scanlon 1998, 113). A person whose desires are rational—not merely that there are eggs in aisle seven, or that the calendar marches forward inevitably—will desire substantive goods. Like Nussbaum, Scanlon is aiming for practical reason to lead us to that which is objectively good, and not merely what an agent happens to desire.

Scanlon does not provide a list of these substantive goods and in fact claims that a degree of flexibility in such an account is called for (Scanlon 1998). At the same time, his "rational aims" criterion prevents him from falling into the subjectivity that would otherwise undermine naïve desire theories. Scanlon claims that a detailed account may be well beyond the level of abstraction of his discussion; his trepidation in laying out the substantive aims of a good life leave the reader with few clues as to what such a life might consist of. At one point he claims that most people have "comprehensive goals of a more modest sort, defined by careers, friendships, marriages and family relations, and political and religious commitments" (Scanlon 1998, 122). Scanlon's discussion of friendship merits being quoted at length:

> A person cannot get the intrinsic benefits of friendship without be-
> ing him- or herself a friend, which involves valuing friendship, that
> is to say, having being a good friend as one of one's aims in the broad
> sense of "aim" that I have been using. A misanthrope, who cares noth-
> ing for friends but to whom others are nonetheless devoted, may
> get some of the instrumental benefits of friendship, such as the help
> that friends provide, but not those benefits that involve standing in
> a certain special relation to others, since he does not stand in that
> relation to anyone. . . . The point is a general one: a life is made better
> by succeeding in one's projects and living up to the values one holds,
> provided these are worthwhile; but if these aims *are* worthwhile then
> succeeding in them will also make one's life better in other ways. This
> is true of friendship because standing in this relation to others is itself
> a good (albeit one that depends on one's having certain aims), and I
> believe that the same can be said of, for example, the achievement of
> various forms of excellence. (Scanlon 1998, 123–124)

Friendships are one of the comprehensive goals that most, although not all people, share. According to Scanlon, the benefits of friendship only accrue to those individuals who are able to be friends to others. Thus, one of the comprehensive goals that most people share involves reciprocal relationships with others. Alvin Goldman makes a similar point about what he calls "social mental interactions [that] influence the quality of life" (Goldman 2006, 298). He points out that many social events (parties, parades, performances) contribute positively to our quality of life precisely because they are shared with other agents, and not merely because of the actual experiences (cocktails and food, victory, music). Being *with* people is better.

Certain claims stand out in Scanlon's discussion. The first is the claim that merely having one's desires fulfilled is not enough for one's life to go well. The second is his claim that there are rational aims that must be fulfilled for a life to be a good human life, in keeping with Nussbaum. His account is not subjectivist, but instead offers a description of a human life that could go well, or go poorly, if certain objectives are not fulfilled. Third, while Scanlon is fairly modest about what these objective criteria might consist in, he offers us some clues as to what those criteria might be, criteria that are primarily relational: marriage, family, religious commitments, and most explicitly, friendships.

Scanlon's discussion goes beyond Warren's in that Scanlon discusses not merely what makes for a member of the moral community, but for a good human life. In so doing, Scanlon makes significant claims about relationships that persons have with other persons. The good life for human beings contains reciprocal relationships.

The implications for persons with theory of mind deficiencies are beginning to emerge. However, a more complete account of Scanlon's "rational aim informed desire" theory is introduced by Veatch. Veatch is a bioethicist looking to answer questions about informed consent and surrogate consent in lieu of direct consent from patients. There are cases in which previously competent patients are not able to make informed decisions about their healthcare, such as cases in which emergency surgery is called for after a serious accident. What course of treatment would a patient choose if he were able to choose? In order of preference, three standards are commonly invoked to solve this problem. The first is that a decision should be made on the basis of the patient's former, explicit wishes. If the patient had a document that laid out his preferences in this case, those instructions should be followed. If no explicit former directives are available, then surrogate decision makers should make decisions on the basis of a substituted judgment, citing what this patient would have consented to were he able to consent in these circumstances. This counterfactual should be resolved by considering the patient's own beliefs and preferences. Finally, if neither of these options presents itself, then surrogate decision makers should make choices based upon a best interest standard, choosing the course of action that would best promote that patient's well-being. The best interest of the patient should encompass the patient's well-being with respect to health, as well as with respect to myriad outcomes that will help contribute to a better course of life. Since there are many cases in which a patient presents in an emergent setting in which there is no clear documentation about what should be done, and in which there is no surrogate present who knows the patient's beliefs and preferences such that a substituted judgment can be employed, health care professionals are often in the position that they must use the best interest standard to determine what should be done for a patient. Thus, a more complete understanding of what a patient's best interest consists in is of significant interest to Veatch.

In order to understand the complexities of the best interest standard, Veatch discusses what well-being might consist in. Veatch adopts a very similar mapping of the kinds of theories that account for well-being as does Scanlon (Veatch 1999). Veatch, like Scanlon, owes much of his discussion to Parfit. The first of these theories is the hedonistic theory: that which makes an agent happiest is that which contributes to well-being. The second is a desire-fulfillment theory, similar to the ones discussed above; the third is an objective list theory. Thus far, given their mutual reliance on Parfit, Scanlon and Veatch share much in common. Of the objective list theory, Veatch remarks "surely there is operating some notion that the good of the patient is objective and external to the patient" (Veatch 1999, 526). Imagine a case in which a head trauma victim was taken to the emergency room without a surrogate present, and the surgeons had to make the decision as to whether to perform one of two procedures. The medical outcomes in this case are clear, but what would the patient want for himself? If the surgeons are told, "Do whatever will make the patient happiest," in keeping with a hedonistic theory, they are given true, but highly impractical advice.

The desire-fulfillment theory is equally uninformative: "Choose the course of action that will help the patient fulfill his desires" may be true, but in these circumstances it is completely unhelpful. The objective list theory presents factual claims about what would contribute to the patient's well-being: "Choose the procedure that will contribute to the patient's ability to engage in his marriage, family, religious commitments, and most explicitly, friendships!" Dr. Scanlon orders. Here the course of action is in keeping with rational aims that in an objective sense all agents would share, if they were operating on informed desires. With this advice the surgeons know which course of action to perform. Only the objective list theory contributes in a substantive way toward answering questions about what the patient would want, and what physicians should do for patients in the absence of patient consent.

Veatch does not present his own list of goods that contribute to well-being, although he cites individuals who have undertaken the project such as Parfit, Bernard Gert and David DeGrazia. Veatch draws some lessons from their work: according to Gert, there is much in common among philosophers' lists of objective goods; according to DeGrazia, spiritual well-being, freedom, and "deep personal relationships" are good for people (Veatch 1999). According to Parfit, some of these goods "might include moral goodness, rational activity, the development of one's abilities, having children and being a good parent, knowledge, and the awareness of true beauty," whereas some of the bad things "might include being betrayed, manipulated, slandered, deceived, being deprived of liberty or dignity, and enjoying either sadistic pleasure, or aesthetic pleasure in what is in fact ugly" (Parfit 1984, 499). There is no complete consensus on what these objective lists might include, and there is some level of subjectivity. Physicians cannot know, in the absence of patient input, the precise preferences or orderings among preferences on each patient's list of objective goods. Ultimately, however, Veatch finds the objective list theory an unsatisfying means by which to employ a best interest standard in clinical decision making, because of the gap between what the clinician knows about the patient and what is in fact objectively in the patient's best interest (Veatch 1999, 526).

Parfit is similarly unwilling to endorse the objective list theory, but for different reasons. Parfit ends his discussion of well-being with the observation that the hedonistic theory without an objective list is misguided, but an objective list without hedonism is unfulfilling for the individual who experiences the so-called objective goods. Thus, what is best for persons is that they experience things that are good, and that they gain genuine enjoyment from those things (Parfit 1984).

Taken together, there are several interesting conclusions to be drawn from the discussions offered by Scanlon, Veatch, and Parfit. The first is that the objective list theories have much to recommend them above experiential/hedonist theories as well as uninformed desire theories of the good, from the point of view of both moral theory and applied ethics. Parfit does not embrace an objective list alone, but recognizes that a hedonistic theory without an objective list is implausible. The second is that philosophers either (a) are loathe to craft precise lists of objective goods, or (b) are sufficiently vague when crafting lists of objective goods so as to render the lists almost—almost—useless. This is Veatch's position, that objective lists may be promising, but what is "objectively in a patient's best interest" may be beyond the treating physician's knowledge (Veatch 1999, 526). Must you be married? Must you have children? Must you have a career or friends? Rarely does a philosopher come down hard on one side, and when he or she does, another philosopher is at the ready to dispute those conclusions. The third conclusion is that despite the vagueness of objective lists, there does seem to be something that they all hold in common: relationships with other human beings are an essential contributor to well-being for humans. Socialization with other humans is so significant that we cannot be said to have well-being without it. No one claims that this socialization must take the shape, for example, of having children. However, well-being requires relationships. It is instructive that Parfit's list of bad states of affairs is concerned predominantly with failures of relationships: betrayals, deceptions, and compromised personal relationships. Thus, a more thorough examination of these relationships should be undertaken.

Hobson on the Human Form of Social Life

Peter Hobson takes up the following question: "What is it to have the human form of social life?" (Hobson 1993, 1). Hobson's concern is not with the intrinsic properties that comprise humanness, or personhood, but rather a question about the types of interactions that one must enter into in order to live a human life. Hobson's position is similar to Kittay's, as she takes issue with "the exclusive use of intrinsic properties in the metaphysics of personhood" (Kittay 2005, 107–108).

Hobson believes that among the essential properties of humans is that humans recognize that other humans have minds and enter into relationships with other humans that reflect this understanding: they participate in "mutual interpersonal transactions," they demonstrate "affective readiness" as well as "understanding of other persons as individualized centres of consciousness with their own psychological orientations towards the world" (Hobson 1993, 1).

According to Hobson, social life "is constituted by relations among persons who understand themselves and others as such" (Hobson 1993, 1); thus, the person lacking theory of mind fails to meet one of the qualities that Hobson considers essential to participate in a human form of social life. At this point it should be observed that Hobson has transitioned from talking about the "human form of social life" to interactions among *persons*. To know what it is for others to be persons, we need to know that we do not treat persons as mere things. Thus, the interrelation between people is an essential part of what it is to know that there actually are other people:

> So in order to know what persons are, one needs to experience and
> understand the kinds of relations that can exist between oneself
> and others—specifically, reciprocal relations based on feelings. For
> instance, an individual would not have an adequate conception of a
> person, if he or she did not know that one cannot always experience
> and treat people as things. (Hobson 1993, 2)

Individuals who miss the concept of what it is to hold particular relations to others are missing out on the human "form of life," as Wittgenstein called it, and thus fail to live a full human life. Hobson uses the example of a man with Asperger's syndrome who was in Hobson's care at one time to illustrate that in order to know what it is to be a friend, one needs to be a friend to others. Sadly, this young man was impassive in his relations with others, unable to be a friend, have friends, or even grasp the concept of a friend, owing to this inability to participate in reciprocal relations with others. Similarly, in order to understand what it is to have the concept of a person, one must stand in the relation of personhood to others. Hobson's position is echoed by Lawson, who takes empathizing, which is not available to the person lacking theory of mind, as the property which "could even be regarded as the factor that makes human society possible" (Lawson 2003, 191).

Hobson goes further than Warren. First, Hobson is not interested merely in what makes an individual a member of the moral community, but he is interested in personhood. Second, it is not merely consciousness, *but consciousness of other persons,* that is essential for personhood. To relate to other persons as if they were objects evidences an inability to recognize what it is for others to be persons. The performance of treating a person like a person is part of the success of recognizing that an individual is a person. It is not sufficient to associate with persons as if they were objects; rather, one must treat them in a particular way. When a person associates with persons but treats them not at all like persons, then there is a sense in which he does not recognize that they *are* persons.

Hobson's focus is not on the cognitive properties, but on the bodily, emotional, and affective aspects of what it is to be person, and in particular what it is to be in contact with other persons. When we take these steps toward others we participate in what Hobson refers to as "reciprocal actions." These actions are affective and moral, but Hobson also believes that these moves toward others have epistemic significance: what it is to know that you are a person, and to recognize other persons *qua* persons, is to reciprocate in this way. This affective reciprocity makes the bodily presence of other persons significant, also. The reciprocal nature of personhood is an embodied experience. This reciprocity allows us to ascribe a directedness of behavior which includes the claim that others have intentions, some of which are understood as propositional attitudes, and that persons' responses to the outside world are in part a condition of the content of their propositional attitudes. Hobson likens the relationship that persons have with other persons to Martin Buber's I-Thou relations, as opposed to the relationship that persons have with objects, which are akin to I-It relationships (Hobson 1993, 5; Buber 2002). A person can have an I-It relationship with the furniture, but *other persons* demand an I-Thou relationship.

Ultimately, the way that we acquire self-knowledge is via knowledge of others; knowledge of others' propositional attitudes allows us to "take the role of the other towards itself" (Hobson 1993, 5). Hobson's position that we come to know ourselves by knowing others is evocative of the TT and ST debate considered in chapter 1. Is theory of mind a mechanism by which we come to know others, the same mechanism by which we come to know ourselves? Even if the *mechanism* is not the same, Hobson is committed to the claim that we do not truly come to know ourselves without knowing others, and vice versa. Echoes of Frith and Happé's arguments about autistic introspection are found in Hobson's account: without an appreciation of other persons as mentalizing beings, the appreciation of ourselves as mentalizing beings is compromised.

Hobson's *question* is the same question asked by Warren: what makes someone a person, a member of the moral community? Hobson's *answer*, however, shares much with claims made by Nussbaum, Scanlon, Veatch, and Parfit about a good human life and well-being: personhood is grounded in relational properties, not intrinsic properties, and in particular in relations that persons have with other persons. Nussbaum, Scanlon, Veatch, and Parfit believe that these relationships are part of what it is for a person's life to *go well,* but according to Hobson, they are not merely about what it is for a person's life to go well, but for an individual to be *a person at all,* that is, a member of the moral community. On Hobson's account, the autistic person fails, due to a lack of theory of mind, to be a member of the moral community. For Hobson, the autistic person is outside the moral community, biologically human but not a person in the moral sense. McGeer cautions against Hobson's approach: ". . . we should be cautious of any account, including Hobson's, that conceptualizes these abnormalities in unilaterally recognitional terms—that is, which emphasizes how the autistic child cannot see us in a certain way because she lacks a theory of mind . . ." (McGeer 2001, 124). McGeer's point is that persons with autism are a mystery to those without autism, but similarly those without autism are a mystery to those with autism. "Some methodological humility is in order," she cautions (McGeer 2001, 127).

If McGeer's words of caution are not heeded, where does that leave the person with autism? One radical answer to this question is presented by Piers Benn.

A Radical View: Benn on Disqualifying Individuals from Membership in the Moral Community

Thus far the discussion has catalogued a set of views about what constitutes moral personhood, a good human life, or membership in the moral community. But few philosophers have moved from these claims to the extreme step of excluding individuals from the moral community. Hobson makes such a claim. Another philosopher who makes this move is Piers Benn.

Benn, like Hobson, considers the relational properties that comprise personhood. Benn's claims mirror Hobson's on the relational and affective aspects of personhood, but Benn does so in the service of excluding individuals, including autistic individuals, from moral consideration (Benn 1999). Benn's work is informed by the work of P. F. Strawson, in particular, Strawson's "Freedom and Resentment" (1974). The following is a version of Benn's argument:

(1) Only those who can possess reactive attitudes can be the object of reactive attitudes;

(2) The autistic person cannot possess reactive attitudes;

(3) Therefore, the autistic person cannot be the object of reactive attitudes;

(4) Only individuals who can possess reactive attitudes and be the object of reactive attitudes are members of the moral community;

(5) Thus, persons with autism are not members of the moral community.

Benn attempts to prove the first premise by citing an example that illustrates the mistake when those who do not possess reactive attitudes become the object of reactive attitudes. In keeping with Strawson, Benn identifies reactive attitudes to be emotions such as anger, frustration, or pride. Benn observes that an agent's anger is appropriately directed only at those who are able to get angry in return. If a hurricane destroys your house, it does not make sense to get angry at the hurricane, because hurricanes do not get angry themselves. Even when agents do get angry at the hurricane, the reasonable agent recognizes the futility and absurdity of doing so. Agents get appropriately angry only at those who are able themselves to experience that emotion; to do otherwise is to make an ontological mistake about the object of reactive attitudes. Benn's justification for this premise is different from Hobson's, but they evidence some similarities. Hobson focuses on reactive attitudes, which he says are the bases for affective relatedness, and not merely rationality or consciousness. Both Hobson and Benn look to the relationships that are part of the objective lists considered by Scanlon, Parfit, and Veatch in an attempt to make further sense of these relationships. For example, Benn notes that when a person is not the kind of person "with whom we can genuinely engage," we cease to hold reactive attitudes toward him (Benn 1999, 31).

The second premise is supported by empirical research on persons with autism. In keeping with the extended quotation from Frith above, deficits in both theory of mind and the ability to mentalize result in a failure of the appropriate response in emotional situations. According to the DSM-IV criteria, persons with autism demonstrate "Qualitative impairments in reciprocal social interaction" (American Psychiatric Association 1994, 70). The person who lacks theory of mind, such that he does not fully ascribe intentional attitudes to others, does not see others as having reactive attitudes. If others do not possess reactive attitudes for the autistic individual, then they are not appropriately the object of reactive attitudes. Similarly, the autistic person, unable to ascribe reactive attitudes to others, does not possess reactive attitudes himself.

The third line of the argument then follows from the first two.

Benn again cites Strawson in defense of the fourth premise: it is inconceivable for us to not participate in "ordinary inter-personal relationships" because to do so is part of the "general framework of human life" (Benn 1999, 30). Individuals who do not participate in such relationships are not members of the moral community. The objective list claim is echoed here, but Benn makes an even stronger point than was made in earlier discussions of objective lists. Previous discussions considered questions about what made a person's life a *good* life: what activities or properties contributed to well-being for a person? Benn's concern is slightly different: what are the activities or properties that contribute to the life of a moral agent at all? Without these properties, one is not merely *a person living a bad life,* but one is *not a person at all,* in the moral sense. Benn's point is not a claim about rationality, although rationality may play an important role in our moral personhood. But reactive attitudes play the most significant role: "whatever reactive attitudes I form about myself, such as pride or guilt, are an inseparable part of my own sense of agency" (Benn 1999, 31). People who do not have these reactive attitudes— children, psychopaths, and persons with autism—are not members of the moral community. Typically developing children who have "the potential to form these attitudes during a normal course of development, as well as the present ability to form them" can nonetheless be treated as members of the moral community; in doing so, children are initiated into the moral community by experiencing adult responses to their reactive attitudes (Benn 1999, 35). Benn acknowledges that there are degrees of psychopathology, and as such, there may be degrees of membership in the moral community. Similarly, perhaps higher-functioning persons with autism, who are able to possess reactive attitudes toward others in virtue of possession of a theory of mind, are members of the moral community. But those who cannot possess reactive attitudes toward others, in light of a compromised theory of mind, are excluded. Just as the hurricane is not a moral agent, in virtue of the fact that it does not possess reactive attitudes, similarly those humans who do not possess reactive attitudes are not moral agents either. Since the person who lacks theory of mind cannot ascribe reactive attitudes, he cannot be the object of reactive attitudes. Thus, he is outside the moral community.

The objections to this argument are best leveled at premise one, premise two, and premise four. Premise one says that it is a mistake to form reactive attitudes toward those who do not themselves possess reactive attitudes. But is this really a mistake? If this is a mistake, then even seemingly rational agents are very often mistaken: people do get angry at the hurricane, or frustrated at the computer, while the hurricane and the computer remain splendidly indifferent. The "pathetic fallacy" is a literary device in which the calm or tumult of nature echoes the calm or turmoil of the characters' inner lives—think of King Lear in the storms or Heathcliff on the shadowy moors. It is a useful literary device, but is a fallacy, and not just in name, to suggest that the weather or other aspects of the environment that lack intentionality are mirroring affective states. The fact that otherwise reasonable agents are often mistaken in their reactive attitudes is not a reason to reject premise one.

An objection to premise two has recently been articulated by David Shoemaker (Shoemaker 2007). Shoemaker proposes a set of necessary and sufficient conditions for moral agency. His view proceeds from P. F. Strawson's and R. Jay Wallace's accounts which hold that the ability to grasp and apply moral reasons, as well the power to act in keeping with such reasons, are the basis of moral agency, a view Shoemaker calls the Moral Reasons-Based Theory of moral agency (MRBT). Shoemaker considers several individuals on the margins of moral agency—the psychopath, the moral fetishist, persons with high-functioning autism, and persons with mental retardation—all of whom occasion a refinement of MRBT. Shoemaker holds that the psychopath and moral fetishist are not moral agents, whereas persons with high-functioning autism and those with mental retardation are. After refining MRBT in light of the above cases, Shoemaker presents the following account of moral agency, one he believes is final and complete:

> MRBT Version 5: One is a member of the moral community, a moral agent eligible for moral responsibility and interpersonal relationships, if and only if (*a*) one has the capacity to recognize and apply second-personal moral reasons one is capable of discovering via identifying empathy with either the affected party (or parties) of one's behavior *or an appropriate representative,* regardless of the method of identification and (*b*) one is capable of being motivated by those

> second-personal moral reasons because one is capable of caring
> about their source (viz., the affected party/parties *or an appropriate*
> *representative*), insofar as one is susceptible to being moved to identi-
> fying empathy with that source by the moral address expressible via
> the reactive attitudes in both its reason-based and emotional aspects.
> (Shoemaker 2007, 107)

Shoemaker brings out two significant points in his analysis. The first concerns his second necessary condition, which requires that moral agents are appropriately motivated by the concerns of others. Here autistic agents succeed where psychopaths do not. Persons with autism can see the concerns of others as motivating factors, while the psychopath remains indifferent to such concerns. But what of Shoemaker's first necessary condition, namely, that moral agents must be able to recognize and apply second-personal moral reasons discovered via identifying empathy, regardless of the method of identification? Understanding this claim requires an explanation of "identifying empathy." Shoemaker claims that "identifying empathy" is "what is involved when we speak of identifying with others: we not only can understand what the world is like for them, but we can also feel what they feel in the way that they feel it. It is this sort of emotional engagement that is at the heart of interpersonal relationships generally, and it is what I call 'identifying empathy'" (Shoemaker 2007, 98–99). Shoemaker holds that the psychopath is incapable of identifying empathy, but the person with high-functioning autism is so capable. Shoemaker grants that the person with autism may be incapable of the simulation theory necessary to understand others' emotional states, but is nonetheless "still capable of the kind of emotional exchange constitutive of moral agency; it's just that the process of getting to the exchange is much more indirect" (Shoemaker 2007, 100). This makes sense of Shoemaker's claim, in part (a) of MRBT Version 5, that a moral agent must be capable of discovering reasons via identifying empathy *regardless of the method of identification*. The person with autism may not be able to undertake these simulations on her own (why is John shivering?), but once the content of others' intentional states is made explicit to her ("Marci, I'm afraid I'll catch a cold but I cannot get up right now to close the window"), then this can be seen as a reason for action (closing the window). This is the basis for Shoemaker's objection to premise two, namely, that the autistic person can possess reactive attitudes, via identifying empathy, even in those cases in which the method of identification may be circuitous.

There are two problems with this view, however. The first is that Shoemaker may be short-changing the hurdles associated with having merely indirect access to others' intentional states. There is a sense, of course, in which every one of us has only indirect access to others' intentional states, but the difficulty for the person with autism in light of theory of mind deficits is particularly challenging. It seems a violation of the moral axiom "ought implies can" to ask of the person with autism to continually perform as a moral agent when these simulations come so hard-won, and in many cases, not at all. Imagine that Marci was autistic. Should she be held morally responsible for her failure to close the window if all she saw was John shivering and his teeth chattering? In the absence of John's explicit request to close the window, we may be asking too much of her. It is, moreover, unclear whether identifying empathy is required at all. If the requirement for moral agency is that others are moved to feel what we feel when we feel it, the bar may be too high for autistic and non-autistic people alike. A second problem is that Shoemaker neither anticipates nor accounts for the unified consciousness view—the view that theory of mind deficits may result in the person with autism falsely believing that everyone else holds the same intentional states that he holds. In this case, the person with autism does apply second-personal moral reasons, but not those discovered via identifying empathy. It would appear that Shoemaker's attempts to respond to the second premise do not adequately take into consideration the significance of theory of mind deficits faced by persons with autism.

Premise four is also problematic. What is the connection between possessing reactive attitudes, being the object of reactive attitudes, and moral agency? Benn claims that reactive attitudes are part of "our own sense of agency" (Benn 1999, 31). The fact that an agent gets angry when he sees an injustice, or that others are rightly angry at him when he perpetuates an injustice, and that he recognizes both of these facts, is part of what it is for him to recognize his own moral agency. This is an *epistemic* claim about an agent's recognition of himself as a moral agent, and not a metaphysical claim about the properties in virtue of which an individual actually has agency. Is Benn claiming that it is impossible to be a moral agent and not be aware of this fact? Perhaps the epistemic and metaphysical points are inextricably linked: an individual's beliefs about his moral obligations are sufficient for that individual to be an agent, and even if that agent is mistaken about those moral obligations, the very fact that the agent has beliefs about moral obligations demonstrate agency.

An objection to this line of reasoning follows from the fact that an agent can have moral responsibilities and not know it. It is possible for an agent to have moral obligations that he fails to recognize. Similarly, might an agent fail to recognize his agency itself? This objection does not seem very convincing. It is true that an agent can have moral obligations that he fails to recognize. But the very fact that an agent can ask himself "Do I have moral obligations?" seems to be sufficient for that agent to have moral obligations. Reflection on the possibility of moral obligations is sufficient for the possession of moral obligations.

The failure of introspection discussed in chapter 1 becomes significant at this point. The failure of theory of mind may compromise not merely an autistic person's ability to come to understand other agents, but it could compromise his ability to come to understand himself. Thus the person with autism might be exactly the individual for whom the question "Do I have moral obligations?" never occurs. If it never occurs to an agent that he has moral obligations, and that agent does not have reactive attitudes, and that agent is not the object of others' reactive attitudes, in what sense is that individual an *agent* at all? This is Benn's point: there are some individuals who are impassive with respect to moral obligations, in virtue of their lack of reactive attitudes.

This failure to appropriately attribute reactive attitudes would not appear *prima facie* sufficient for a failure of agency. Aristotle, for example, recognized the moral importance of anger. When an injustice occurs Aristotle claims that it is important to get angry, and to get angry in the right way: toward the right people, to the right extent at the right time, for the right reasons (Aristotle 1955, 1109a27). Implicit in this claim is the notion that we can fail to get angry in the right ways.

One of these failures would be to never get angry at all. That Erin does not get angry at an injustice does not exempt her from moral agency; rather, for Aristotle, Erin may well be a moral agent who has simply failed in her obligations. The fact that a person does not have reactive attitudes toward others does not exempt her from moral agency. Perhaps it is not the attribution of reactive attitudes to others that makes one a moral agent, but the fact that *others appropriately possess reactive attitudes toward an individual* which makes that individual a moral agent. It is possible for Erin to be the appropriate object of reactive attitudes. If it is possible to rightly get angry at Erin when she fails to act morally, and she is appropriately the object of such a reactive attitude, then she qualifies as a moral agent. Erin is a moral agent, but the hurricane is not, precisely because it is possible for others to appropriately get angry at Erin, but not at the hurricane. The reason this sounds true is that it is, but it is also question-begging. If a person can rightly be held morally responsible, then he is the kind of person who can have moral responsibilities. Has Benn told us anything we do not already know?

Perhaps he has, in that Benn does not merely claim that the person with autism who cannot possess reactive attitudes does not have moral responsibilities, but that *non-autistic people do not have moral responsibilities toward them.* Moral agents owe something to Erin, insofar as she can both possess and be the object of reactive attitudes. No one morally owes the hurricane anything, in light of the hurricane's lack of reactive attitudes. Warren claims that those outside of the moral community do not have full moral rights. Benn goes further than Warren in stating that agents do not have moral obligations to the autistic individual, as he stands outside the moral community. Benn's claims are both about what the autistic person owes us, and what we owe the autistic person. Owing to a lack of reciprocity, both answers are the same: nothing at all.

Refuting the Radical View:
What Is Lost When Others Are Excluded

Psychiatric disorders are those in which person and syndrome
are most confusingly entwined; the clinical challenge is to tease
out and nurture the moral agent within the syndrome, to preserve
the patient's autonomous personhood. Psychiatry is therefore
an irreducibly moral enterprise, and disagreements about what
constitutes "true" personhood give rise to a number of professional
controversies. (Scheurich 2002, 15)

Reciprocity cuts both ways. Benn's dismissal of the autistic person
from moral consideration does not only cut the autistic person off
from non-autistic, but cuts the non-autistic off from autistic persons.
If this loss of reciprocity is devastating to the autistic person, so too
will it be devastating to the non-autistic person (Adshead 1999). What
is lost when humans distance themselves from others by removing
them from moral consideration? The ills of exclusion emerge on two
levels. First, the performance of morally wrong actions can result from
these attitudes. Second, there is an erosion of the moral status of the
autistic and non-autistic person alike when any persons are excluded
from moral consideration.

Historically, tremendous injustices are perpetrated when some
humans make the claim that other humans are less than persons, or
not as deserving of moral consideration. Two familiar examples are the
Nazi Holocaust, in which Jews, Gypsies, and others were slaughtered
on the basis of the belief that they did not merit full moral consideration, and the eugenics movement in the United States, in which
tens of thousands of people were forcibly sterilized on the basis of the
belief that they were "feeble-minded" or carried some other defect.
The belief that some humans deserve less-than-full status in the moral
community can lead to actions with horrific consequences.

But what if none of these injustices were perpetuated, and it was
merely the case that those perceived as non-members of the moral
community were allowed to live out their lives in a separate, but parallel, world? None of the horrific consequences need occur, and instead, a benign moral indifference could reign. Humans who were not

considered part of the moral community could be cared for, even as their status as outside the moral community was affirmed by others. Especially from a consequentialist standpoint, nothing would be lost under these circumstances.

However, even within the framework of benign moral indifference, a second ill of moral exclusion emerges: *agents compromise their own moral standing,* their own claim to membership in the moral community, when they disqualify others. In chapter 1, McGeer is noted that the non-autistic person's inability to "get" persons with autism is on par with the autistic person's inability to "get" those without autism. By shutting out the person with autism, those who are not autistic shut themselves out as well. The moral standing of anyone is damaged whenever that person affirms that some other human being is disqualified from moral consideration. The non-autistic person who exempts the autistic person on the basis a perceived lack of ability to enter into reciprocal relationships eliminates reciprocal relationships with autistic persons out-of-hand. The very basis upon which the non-autistic person excludes the autistic person becomes the basis upon which the non-autistic person ultimately excludes himself. We should continue to be as inclusive as possible when determining who should count as a member of the moral community, because the costs are so high if we are wrong.

An objection to this position may be that it is a rather selfish justification for inclusion: include others, lest you place yourself in moral danger. It is true that this is a selfish argument for inclusion, but why is that an objection? Selfish motives may be among the most intractable. Selfishness may not be the most attractive basis upon which to build a claim about the moral status of others, but none is more solid. One examination of motives is presented by Thomas H. Murray. In his discussion of why parents have children, Murray divides motivations into those which are selfish, those which are based on altruism, and what he refers to as "mutualism" (Murray 1996). Selfish motives are "commonly regarded as either morally neutral or bad, but robust and reliable," whereas altruism is "more morally reputable, but not as robust" (Murray 1996, 62). Mutualism, which promotes fulfillment between both the parent and the child, is a third way that Murray finds most acceptable. But mutualism is not available when considering persons with autism. So mutualism is not available as a motive to include persons with autism in the moral community. The assumptions behind mutualism, such as "with the support of appropriate social institutions and practices, relationships characterized by mutuality can and do exist" (Murray 1996, 62), do not hold for persons with autism. But Murray is right—altruism is too precarious a foundation upon which to build something so significant as the moral claims of persons. Thus, selfishness is the best option available.

This position should be distinguished from one that is commonly held, that otherwise healthy people "have so much to learn" from persons with disabilities, or that persons with disabilities can teach those without disabilities about love, or caring, or what really matters in life. This view is akin to a "soul-making" view, as it has passing similarity with John Hick's theodicy. Hick holds that evil persists in a world inhabited by an omnibenevolent God because evil helps humans to become better people: evil helps to improve our souls (Hick 1977, 261). In a similar fashion to the soul-making view, disabilities such as autism help to make those who care for persons with autism better people. The problem with the soul-making view is that it still relegates persons with disabilities to a lesser status. On the soul-making view, a person with autism has a paltry supporting role in the life story of healthy protagonists who come to acquire a richer understanding of the world thanks to the participation of an autistic person in their lives. Unquestionably, this falls far short of treating a person with autism as a moral equal. Persons with autism should not be used merely as a means of character development for non-autistic persons. Rather, both autistic and non-autistic persons must be perceived as full members of the moral community, because exclusion of one will impair the moral status of the other.

A second objection can be made to the claim that persons with autism should have full moral status because of the harm that accrues to non-autistic persons when they are not accorded full moral status. According full moral status to persons with autism on the basis of the fact that *persons without autism are harmed by treating persons with autism in a particular way*, is really not that different from the soul-making view, which holds that *persons without autism are benefited by treating persons with autism in a particular way.* Is not the view that persons with autism should be accorded full moral status because of the harm to non-autistic persons just as demeaning as the soul-making view? It is not, for two reasons. First, on the soul-making view, non-autistic persons are better off *because* some persons lack Nussbaum's human capabilities, or the properties that are required for Scanlon's, Parfit's, and Veatch's well-being. The cost to improve the lives of non-autistic persons comes at the expense of persons with autism on the soul-making view. But the harms of *not* excluding others from moral status can be avoided at no one's expense. Second, the two views are dissimilar because the position advocated here is one that results in *all* persons having full moral status. On the soul-making view, there are winners and losers, star players with full moral status, and the supporting cast there to make the stars (look) good. The non-altruistic motive to include autistic persons in the moral community may be selfish, but doing so does not come at a moral cost to autistic community.

Exclusion of others from the moral community is not an option, but the possibility of a moral theory that can be shared across the experiences of both autistic and non-autistic people alike is not promising. The next chapter examines the complexities in finding a theory that governs the moral status of actions which can be shared across the divide that separates us.

Voices of Autism

Gunilla Gerland's autobiography, A Real Person, focuses primarily on her childhood and early adulthood in Sweden. Only as an adult was she finally diagnosed with autism. Her failure to fit in as a child was chalked up to "defiance," rather than the profound difficulties she faced. She was plagued by the realization that she was different from other children, and harbored a deep desire to be like everyone else. Her sister, Kerstin, was one of the few children with whom Gunilla could play as a young child, because Kerstin and Gunilla's games were informed by rule, ritual, and consistency. Gunilla took everything that people said around her literally, assuming, for example, that others could see into the future when they asserted, "You're going to like going to school." But school was filled with scores of children with "empty faces" whom Gerland could only occasionally remember, and even more rarely, understand. Her adolescence was marred by her father's abandonment of the family, as well as her mother's descent into alcoholism and mental illness.

Gerland describes the failure to recognize the moral import of actions and events around her. A variety of stories capture this confusion. In one, she tells of her sister's lack of interest in playing the game "cars," and the bribes that she had to pay Kerstin to induce her to play. Gerland paid the bribes by stealing from her mother, saying, "I didn't mind doing that at all" (Gerland 1996, 38). In another episode, she recounts her father's first abandonment of their family when she was four and a half. Her mother took in boarders after he left, which necessitated rearranging the rooms in the house. Gerland was unperturbed by the loss of her father, comparing his departure to a bowl of fruit that was on the table one day and gone the next. "On the other hand, it greatly disturbed me when they moved the furniture," she writes (Gerland 1996, 42–43).

School posed equal challenges to Gerland's moral assessment of actions. She was routinely taken to the lavatories at her school and punched in the stomach by some of the boys. This went on for some time until another student disclosed this harassment to a teacher who made the boys stop. Gerland was upset that she was manipulated by the boys, and upset that the teacher put an end to the maltreatment: "It was now quite clear that I had been deceived in some way, so I felt stupid. Hadn't I gone and found those boys myself, in case on some days they had forgotten to hit me?" (Gerland 1996, 92).

Gerland continues to be confronted with similar challenges in adult life. Unlike people who are not autistic, Gerland finds that she is ". . . unable to perceive whether people wish me well or ill. I try to calculate with my intellect, and the result is not always that good" (Gerland 1996, 244). In addition to complicating her relationships with other people, autism has affected Gerland's ability to make sense of the moral landscape.

3

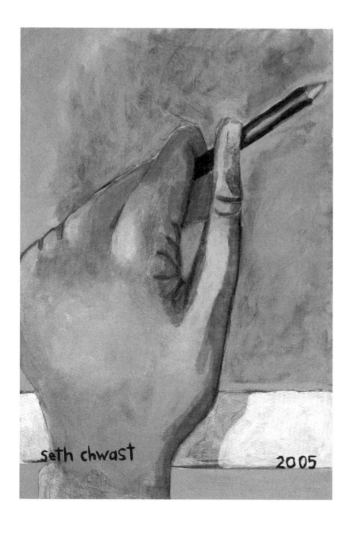

SETH CHWAST, *HAND HOLDING THE PENCIL*

Autism and Moral Theories

The previous chapter considered the moral status of the person with autism. What role does the person with autism have in the moral community, given that he is cut off from other persons in a fundamental way, and what do theories about well-lived human lives tell us about the lives of persons with autism? These questions are precursors to questions about what persons who do not have autism morally owe those who do, and what individuals with autism can reasonably be expected to owe those without autism. Questions about what we owe other persons, and what they owe us, are answered by moral theories that consider the rightness and wrongness of actions. Thus, an investigation of the applicability of different moral theories to the autistic individual is the next step in an inquiry into the ethics of autism.

Can autistic individuals have a moral sense at all? Should we speak of moral theories' applicability to individuals who do not recognize moral dilemmas, and cannot distinguish moral questions from other types of questions? Given that ought implies can, if autistic individuals are not able to recognize moral questions when confronted with them, then autistic individuals cannot be required to act in keeping with any moral theory. Two types of evidence present themselves in favor of the claim that some autistic individuals do have a moral sense. The first is anecdotal evidence: plenty of autistic individuals evidence moral concerns. The anecdotal evidence—being anecdotal, after all—is too wide-ranging to systematically categorize. Frith, for example, cites examples of persons with autism who are recognized as not merely having a strong moral sense, but in some cases were recognized as moral exemplars. Frith recounts stories of the twelfth-century

Franciscan monk, Brother Juniper, a historical figure who seemed to have many traits associated with autism, but who was also recognized as a paradigm of piety, humility, and selflessness (Frith 2003).

Second, at least two studies support the claim that persons with autism do make moral distinctions. One study was conducted by R. James R. Blair (Blair 1996). Blair ran an experiment with four groups of ten children each: ten typically developing children, ten with moderate learning difficulties, ten children with autism who were able to pass two false-belief tests, and ten children with autism unable to pass the two false-belief tests. Blair's experiment involved presenting the children with a set of vignettes, to see if the children could tease out the distinction between violating moral transgressions, such as "a child hitting another child," and what Blair described as "conventional" transgressions, such as "a boy child wearing a skirt" (Blair 1996, 572). Blair found that "the children with autism made a distinction between moral and conventional transgressions in their judgments . . . [and] that the level of ability on false-belief tasks is not associated with the tendency to distinguish moral and conventional transgressions; even the least able of the groups of children with autism were recognizing the moral/conventional distinction" (Blair 1996, 577). Psychologists may be unsatisfied with the study because it was comparatively small; philosophers may be unsatisfied with the moral/conventional distinction, as well as the examples that were used to illustrate the distinction.[1] In a second study, Cathy M. Grant, Jill Boucher, Kevin J. Riggs, and Andrew Grayson compared a group of nineteen children with autism spectrum disorders (seventeen with autism, two with Asperger's syndrome), seventeen children with "moderate learning difficulties" (MLD), and a typically developing control group on both judgments of moral culpability as well as justifications for those judgments (Grant et al. 2005). The children in the study were given six pairs of vignettes, and were asked of the agents in each story, "Which one of these two children is the naughtier?" After receiving the answer, the study subjects were then asked, "Why? Why do you think that X is the naughtier?" Grant et al. examined whether children with autism were more inclined to make moral judgments on the basis of agents' motives or on the basis of the consequences of actions, as well as whether children with autism were more inclined to view harms to other persons as more significant than harms to non-persons. Grant et al. found that "All [three of] the groups based their judgments on the motive of the protagonist" (Grant et al. 2005, 322), favoring deontological intuitions over consequentialist ones. Further, "All three groups judged damage to people to be more serious than damage to property" (Grant et al. 2005, 322). However, when presenting the three groups with more complex pairs of vignettes, "The typically developing group scored at ceiling . . . always judging on the basis of the protagonist's motive. In comparison, the autism and MLD groups under-performed on this task compared to the typically developing group" (Grant et al. 2005, 322).[2] Grant et al. found all three groups comparably poor in their ability to offer justifications for the wrongness of agents' actions. Grant et al. cite Blair's observation about moral rules and social-conventional rules, suggesting that this distinction may also account for children with autism's judgment that harming a person is more blameworthy than harming property. However, Grant et al. also suggest that "a simpler explanation may be that the children with autism who we tested have been explicitly taught that damage to people is more culpable than to objects or property" (Grant et al. 2005, 326). *Do not hit your brother* is doubtless stressed more often, with more force, and with greater sanction if violated than *do not hit your teddy bear*. Finally, Grant et al. hypothesize that executive function impairments may account for autistic children's inability to offer appropriate justifications of moral culpability. As with Blair's study, this study was somewhat small.

Until further evidence is gathered, both Blair's and Grant et al.'s studies are among the few that attempt to locate—and in fact do locate—a moral sense in persons with autism. It makes sense to conclude that some persons with autism recognize moral questions, just as some persons in the non-autistic population can recognize moral questions. The next step is to locate a moral theory suited to both autistic and non-autistic persons alike.

Given unique deficits faced by persons with autism, it appears that many well-regarded moral theories will fail to be applicable to autistic moral agents. The discussion is not meant to be a discussion about which moral theory is true; rather, the consideration is which moral theory is workable, practical, and able to be effectively implemented by both autistic and non-autistic persons alike. Consider a thought experiment: imagine that there was a true moral theory, but it was definitionally beyond the ability of any person to know what that theory claimed. Perhaps it was a deontological moral theory whose rules could never be exhaustively determined. A fact of the matter existed about the rightness or wrongness of given actions, but that fact was forever out of the reach of moral agents. Such a theory could not be objected to on the basis of its falsehood. Instead, the theory's impracticality would be of significant concern. The theory would violate the moral axiom that ought implies can, as moral agents would be obligated to adhere to a set of rules that they could not recognize. As with some of the children in Grant et al.'s study, if some of the justifications for what counts as a morally right or wrong action are beyond autistic agents' abilities to either understand or implement, the moral theory that determines rightness and wrongness would not be practical. In similar fashion, the chapter examines the limits of some moral theories for autistic agents, showing that the nature of these theories renders them unworkable for autistic agents.

This chapter presents a few prominent theories that would be most profoundly challenged by the autistic agent. Is the inability to enter into relationships with other persons *qua* persons, or the inability to feel a certain type of empathy, grounds for rejecting some moral theories? Do other difficulties that the person with autism faces, such as lack of imaginative play, or weak central coherence, bear on the applicability of certain moral theories? The autistic person is still owed moral obligations, as Nussbaum observes, but which moral theories bridge the gap between autistic and non-autistic individuals? Nussbaum observes that philosophers are mistaken when they conflate the questions "By whom are society's basic principles designated?" and "For whom are society's basic principles designated?" (Nussbaum 2006). Nussbaum's focus is on the limits of social contract theories and other theories of justice, but her point is also applicable to normative theories about the rightness and wrongness of actions. But what of individuals who do have sufficient agency to act according to some normative theory's prescriptions, but over whom the theories have no sway? The attempt by Benn to disqualify the autistic person from moral consideration comes at too high a cost. The next step is to consider which normative theories are available to govern conduct among autistic and non-autistic persons.

The first moral theory examined is David Hume's, which relies heavily on feelings of sympathy shared among members of the moral community. Jeanette Kennett argues that Hume's moral theory is not available to the autistic individual. (While this section of the chapter focuses on Hume's theory, it also includes a brief aside examining the shortcomings of utilitarian theories.) Kennett claims that the autistic individual is on safer ground adopting Immanuel Kant's moral theory. Thus, Kantian moral theory is discussed second. While there are some aspects of Kantian moral theory that prove attractive for autistic moral agents, some formulations of the categorical imperative are not as promising. Benn dismisses a Kantian social contract theory as not open to the autistic individual. After examining Kantian moral theory, the chapter explores both moral particularism and an ethic of *prima facie* duties. Moral particularism does not seem to hold promise for autistic individuals. John Lawson dismisses an ethic of *prima facie* duties as unworkable for the autistic individual. There is a divide between the moral theories available to the autistic person and the non-autistic person, and it is not clear how to bridge this gap. The chapter closes with an applied question that is raised by this divide: if a means to "cure" adults with autism is found, who makes the choice to apply it? The difficulties in answering this question illustrate the complexities of finding common moral ground between autistic and non-autistic individuals.

A final note: each of these theories has its own proponents and critics. Rather than present a comprehensive account of all of the objections to each theory, the question at hand is how the theories are challenged by the notion of autistic moral agents. There may be reasons for rejecting one, or all, of the theories considered that have nothing to do with persons with autism. The immediate project, however, is to show how autism in particular presents a novel challenge to these ethical theories.

Kennett: A Rejection of Humean Theories

Kennett argues that Humean moral theory is not available to the autistic individual. Understanding Kennett's argument first requires a brief discussion of Hume's moral theory, and then a discussion of the autistic individual's unique characteristics that make it impossible for him to employ Hume's moral theory.

According to Hume's moral theory a feeling of sympathy is required for morality. Hume observes that reason, in the form of impressions or ideas, "can never produce any action or give rise to volition," nor can reason prevent actions or volitions (Hume 1948, 24). Rather, passion is what directs our actions, and since actions are the kinds of things that are moral or immoral, it is passions, and not reason, that determine morality:

> Since morals, therefore, have an influence on the actions and affections, it follows that they cannot be derived from reason, and that because reason alone, as we have already proved, can never have any such influence. Morals excite passions, and produce or prevent actions. Reason of itself is utterly impotent in this particular. The rules of morality, therefore, are not conclusions of our reason. (Hume 1948, 33)

According to Hume, morality is "more felt than judged of" (Hume 1948, 43), and "morality is determined by sentiment" (Hume 1948, 265). One emotion in particular, sympathy, is at the center of Hume's moral theory. According to Kennett, sympathy is necessary for moral agency on Hume's account. Sympathy is gained by mirroring other people: "It seems that one learns about and develops one's own mental states in concert with others" (Kennett 2002, 343). An interesting implication of this is that it is not merely the case that what we know of others we learn via an understanding of ourselves, but what we know of ourselves we know via an understanding of others in keeping with both the dialectical understanding of autism (Stanghellini 2001) and Frith and Happé's claims about autism and self-consciousness.

Kennett echoes Adshead in her description of empathy as "the capacity to form the other-regarding beliefs which are central to recognizable moral thought"; elsewhere Kennett says, "empathy involves, or is underwritten by, a capacity to enter sympathetically into the concerns and feelings of others" (Kennett 2002, 341). As stated in chapter 1, empathy is at odds with a unified consciousness view. The unified consciousness view is the belief that all agents have the same intentional states. On this view, there is a limited call for empathy—other-regarding beliefs—because those beliefs are identical to those an agent holds himself. Imagine that both John and Marci desire the window closed in the cold room. She feels just as cold as he does, and can feel bad that he is equally uncomfortable, but hers is a slim type of empathy if it only emerges when she experiences the same intentions as John. Thus, empathy requires both the recognition that other agents have intentional states, and the recognition that some states are distinct from an agent's own intentional states. In chapter 2, Frith was quoted at length describing intentional empathy, the ability to understand another's reasons for an emotional response, and the ability to form an appropriate response to another's emotional state. It would appear that by "sympathy," Hume means what we mean by "empathy." The crucial difference between these two accounts of empathy—the notion of other-regarding beliefs on one hand, and the notion of sympathy for the concerns and the feelings of others, on the other hand—is that the first requires the empathetic person to *form* beliefs *about* others, whereas the second requires the empathetic person to *recognize the beliefs possessed by others*.[3] The first account does not pose a difficulty for persons with autism—it is possible to form a belief about others without having a full-fledged theory of mind. But the second account, in which the empathetic person ascribes beliefs to others, may pose a significant challenge to the person lacking theory of mind. Given the role of sympathy/empathy in Hume's moral theory, questions can now be raised as to whether the autistic individual is able to be a Humean. Three reasons can be offered for thinking that the autistic individual is unable to experience empathy, and thus is unable to employ Hume's moral theory. The first focuses on theory of mind deficits, the second considers philosophy of language and the autistic speaker, and the third examines the implications of the TT versus ST debate to Humean moral theory.

A first piece of evidence for the claim that persons with autism are unable to experience empathy is the difficulty theory of mind poses for many autistic individuals.[4] Here the difference between the two accounts of empathy emerges: the individual who does not ascribe false beliefs to others, and thus may not ascribe beliefs to others, may nonetheless form other-regarding beliefs. The first sense of "empathy" is unchallenged by false-belief tasks and their implications for theory of mind. The second sense of "empathy," however, provides a greater challenge. It does not make sense to say that an individual who lacks theory of mind understands the concerns and feelings of others. Persons who, in virtue of their own impoverished theory of mind, do not have a rich conception of other persons as having minds cannot be empathetic toward other persons. Kennett also cites the lack of imaginative play on the part of autistic individuals as evidencing an inability of autistic persons to place themselves in the position of others (Kennett 2002, 346), echoing Neil Scheurich who observes that "the project of empathy . . . is fundamentally an act of imagination" (Scheurich 2002, 17). Lack of imaginative play is cited as a reason to believe that children with autism lack theory of mind (Baron-Cohen 1995, 76–77; Gopnik et al. 2000, 61; Siegel 1998, 64). Lack of imaginative play also bespeaks a failure of the mirroring that characterizes the dialectical conception of autism. Persons with autism are unable to exercise empathy in part because they do not really know other people, and in part because they do not really know themselves, in keeping with Happé and Frith's observations in chapter 1. Taken together, these claims about the lack of theory of mind point to the failure of persons with autism to exercise empathy toward others. Kennett says that she is interested in those persons with autism who do evidence theory of mind, and are able to pass false-belief tests, but who nonetheless "still find simulation of the mental states, and in particular the moods and intentions of others, very difficult or unreliable" (Kennett 2002, 345–346). For such persons, the notion of empathy would be difficult; *a fortiori,* consistent and effortless empathy would be impossible.

Kennett cites impaired language ability, especially with respect to pragmatics, in the case of higher-functioning persons with autism as evidence of an individual's inability to understand and empathize with others (Baron-Cohen 1995; Glüer and Pagin 2003). "The autistic speaker is also characterized by his lack of understanding or concern for the interpretational needs and abilities of the interlocutor" (Glüer and Pagin 2003, 30). Unlike non-native speakers, or other individuals who are just developing a facility with a given language, many autistic individuals never master the pragmatics of language. As discussed in chapter 1, pragmatics are intimately tied to empathy, in that grasping the pragmatics of a language involves understanding, appreciating, and compensating for what others do not understand.

The final, and most elaborate, discussion on Kennett's part concerns the inability of persons with autism to employ either TT or ST, each of which evidences an inability to place oneself in others' shoes. As discussed in chapter 1, TT and ST are competing theories about the explanation of human action. When John gets up out of his chair, crosses the room, closes the window, and sits back down, Marci may cite two possible theories to explain John's behavior. The first is to cite TT: Marci ascribes intentionality to John, including beliefs about the draftiness of the room, or desires to quell the noise from the neighbor's house. In the case of TT, Marci makes intentional ascriptions about John—a process of explanation not open to the person who lacks theory of mind. The second theory that Marci might use to explain John's behavior is ST: Marci does not directly ascribe intentionality to John, but rather makes a claim about *her* intentions were she in John's position, which would cause her to close the window. Marci then explains John's behavior by reference to a counterfactual: "If I were to get up from being seated in that room and close the window, only to sit back down, then I would be responding to the horrible draft. That explains John's behavior, too." Kennett contends that empathetic approaches are closely tied to simulation. She compares the process of Humean sympathy to R. M. Hare's third-stage universalizability, in which we imagine what it is to occupy others' positions, and we "cannot keep these simulations off line" (Kennett 2002, 344).[5] Hare then goes further, by claiming that the fact that this move is mandatory leads to the inevitability that we will "catch" the desires we simulate: for Marci to employ ST in explaining John's closing of the window is for her to empathize with what it means to be sitting uncomfortably in a cold room. If an agent does not understand the desire sufficiently to "catch" it, perhaps the agent never understood it in the first place. Goldman says that merely "catching" an attitude is insufficient for moral consideration—catching is merely a lower level of simulation. A second step is required: there must be a "concern mechanism" by which persons are *themselves* affected by the concerns of *others*. Goldman cites Shaun Nichols who hypothesizes that psychopaths have an intact lower level of simulation, and are in fact often very aware of others' affective states, but simply do not care about those states, in contrast to the autistic. Persons with autism "have impaired perspective-taking abilities but an intact concern mechanism. Psychopaths, by contrast, have a normal capacity for perspective taking but a deficit in the concern mechanism" (Goldman 2006, 293). As discussed in chapter 1, if Marci were autistic she might not be able to use either TT or ST to know why John wanted the window closed, but once presented with those facts, she would likely show concern and empathy. But owing to theory of mind deficits, Marci is not an empathy self-starter—her concern would only emerge once John's circumstances were made explicit to her. The psychopathic Marci would not evidence concern, even when John's discomfort was made explicit to her. An agent who is indifferent to the suffering of others cannot be said to truly understand that suffering—again, it is a slim "sympathy" that takes stock of the suffering of others, but does so with indifference. The simulation that is undertaken when an agent exercises Humean sympathy requires an agent to "experience real, if second-hand, emotion" (Kennett 2002, 344).

Karsten R. Stueber makes a distinction between two types of empathy. The first, which he calls "basic empathy," is the mechanism that allows agents to recognize that a person is angry or that he is about to grasp a cup; the second, called "reenactive empathy," is "using our cognitive and deliberative capacities in order to reenact or imitate in our own mind that thought processes of the other person" (Stueber 2006, 21). This reenactive empathy requires Marci to not merely recognize John's discomfort, but to experience some discomfort herself. She does not necessarily get goose bumps on her arm or shiver at the cold, but she does feel something for John upon recognizing his discomfort. The inability of Marci to form real, albeit secondhand, emotions has much in common with Gopnik et al.'s discussion of the failure of theory formation, not a failure of theory of mind per se, in autism (Gopnik et al. 2000). Gopnik et al.'s position was articulated in chapter 1: perhaps there is no explicit theory of mind module, but rather, a general process of theory formation, which is incapacitated in individuals with autism. This accounts for a failure to successfully apply either TT or ST. Gopnik et al. recount an experimental result: "It is of special interest that for the autistic children there was a correlation between an individual child's imitation score and how well that child responded on [a] test of empathy" (Gopnik et al. 2000, 61). Even if theory of mind is impeded due to a general failure of theory formation, the results are the same.

In addition to the evidence from the psychological literature, there is also evidence for these claims from the physiological research. A small, post-mortem study found that men with autism had fewer cells in their amygdala—the portion of the brain that processes emotions (Schumann and Amaral 2006). This observation is not sufficient to determine if fewer cells result in more limited social experiences, or if more limited social experiences cause a reduction in the number of cells, however (Khamsi 2006).

While the physiological evidence is inconclusive, the evidence from psychological tests shows that autistic individuals are often unable to undertake the imaginative shift that would allow them to form the counterfactual about others' intentions that are distinct from their own, a step which is essential to employing ST. An example of the failure of an autistic person to exercise simulation is presented by Kennett. A teenager with autism named Jack was tremendously bothered by the notion that some homes lack perfectly tuned pianos, to the point that he suggested a constitutional amendment be adopted to remedy the situation. Jack was unable to suspend his own beliefs and preferences sufficiently so as to simulate what it would be like to be someone who was indifferent to the condition of the ill-tuned piano:

> Able autistic people may attempt to run simulations of other people's mental states in developing the rules, or in applying them in particular cases; but like Jack they run into problems, since they do not have

the capacity to imagine responses which differ from their own. Simulation is not a reliable way for autistic people to get the information they need to arrive at a judgment. (Kennett 2002, 351)

Imagine that Marci has autism. If Marci is not the kind of person who is bothered by a draft, then she may have difficulty in imagining that John would be bothered by drafts, resulting in an inability to apply ST correctly—"In real empathy, as opposed to mere emotional contagion, the empathizer has to recognize that the other person is in distress and needs comfort, even if they are not in the same distress themselves" (Gopnik et al. 2000, 56). This is why Goldman refers to ST as "the empathy theory" (Goldman 2006, 11). In cases in which empathetic thinking is a crucial element in making a correct judgment, the autistic person who relies on ST will fall short. Sympathy involves simulating the intentions of others. Thus any moral theory that relies heavily on the notion of sympathy will not be available to the person with autism. An alternative interpretation of Jack's position emerges from the unified consciousness view. Perhaps Jack does recognize that other persons have intentional states, but is unable to distinguish those intentional states from his own. The consequence, however, is the same: either a failure of ST owing to theory of mind deficits or a unified consciousness view will result in a failure of empathy on Jack's part.

The deficits faced by the autistic person result in a lack of empathy, the consequences of which are "moral indifference" (Kennett 2002, 342). A lack of theory of mind may leave an individual in a state of skepticism or state of inquiry (Minkowski and Targowla 2001), but not a state of empathy. Without this feeling, an agent would be unable to act rightly or wrongly according to Hume's moral theory. Thus, Hume's moral theory is not applicable to the person with autism.

The lack of sympathy on the part of the autistic person also poses a challenge, albeit an indirect one, to a classical version of utilitarianism. John Stuart Mill, in chapter 3 of *Utilitarianism*, discusses what he calls "the ultimate sanction of the principle of utility" (Mill 1979, 26). This ultimate sanction is the motivating factor that compels each of us to be utilitarians. Mill's utilitarianism requires agents to perform those actions that promote the greatest balance of pleasure over pain for all parties affected by those actions. Furthermore, all individuals should be taken into account equally: social proximity does not matter, only the total amount of pleasure and pain. Given the self-sacrificing nature of utilitarianism, it is incumbent upon the utilitarian to argue for the appeal of his theory, which is why Mill devotes considerable discussion to the question of sanctions. Mill divides sanctions into two types: those external to the agent, and those internal to the agent. While it is problematic to divide motivating factors into those that come from outside of an agent, and those that come from within—is "peer pressure" an external or internal motivator?—this difficulty is not of immediate concern when examining the challenge autistic agents pose to utilitarianism. Of external sanctions, Mill refers to the "hope of favor and fear of displeasure from our fellow creatures or from the Ruler of the universe, along with whatever we may have of sympathy or affection for them, or of love and awe of Him, inclining us to do His will independently of selfish consequences" (Mill 1979, 27). In addition to these external sanctions, there is a single internal sanction:

> The internal sanction of duty, whatever our standard of duty may be, is one and the same—a feeling in our own mind; a pain, more or less intense, attendant on violation of duty, which in properly cultivated moral natures rises, in the more serious cases, into shrinking from it as an impossibility. This feeling, when disinterested and connecting itself with the pure idea of duty, and not with some particular form of it, or with any of the merely accessory circumstances, is the essence of conscience; though in that complex phenomena as it actually exists, the simple fact is in general all encrusted over with collateral associations derived from sympathy, from love, and still more from fear; from all the forms of religious feeling; from the recollections of childhood and of all our past life; from self-esteem, desire of the esteem of others, and occasionally even self-abasement. (Mill 1979, 28)

The internal sanction is a feeling of guilt, conscience, or remorse upon the recognition that we have failed in our duties to others, duties that we acknowledge from our youngest days, and which emerge from deep feelings of sympathy, love, and fear. Sympathy is significant in motivating us to be utilitarians: without a feeling of sympathy for our fellow creatures, we have neither external nor internal motivation to maximize utility, especially when such maximizing comes at a cost to ourselves. Those who do not have the appropriate feelings of sympathy will not find a persuasive reason to practice utilitarianism.

It is not clear that the failure of the ultimate sanction is a crushing blow to the utilitarian. A moral theory may be true, even if agents are not sufficiently motivated to act in keeping with the theory. The truth of a theory may not be sufficient for agents to act according to the theory's guidelines. But in addition to being true, a moral theory should also be practical, and without sanction, it is not clear that utilitarianism meets this requirement. Thus, the lack of sympathy on the part of the autistic individual does pose a problem for the utilitarian,[6] as well as the Humean.

In reply to the autistic agent's challenge to Humean ethics, there are three responses. First, it is possible that the feelings of sympathy and empathy refer to different concepts; thus, while the autistic person lacks empathy, this lack does not pose a direct challenge to Hume's theory. The second claims that given Humean moral theory the autistic person cannot act morally, and simply acknowledges that the autistic person is somehow beyond moral agency. The third concedes that the autistic person does pose a significant challenge to Humean ethics, and that another moral theory merits consideration.

The first response, that Humean sympathy and the contemporary notion of empathy are different concepts, is not promising. The distinction between sympathy and empathy is often made in the following manner: sympathy involves feelings *toward* another, whereas empathy involves feeling *as* another feels. Marci feels sympathy when she feels bad for the fact that John is uncomfortable; she feels empathy when, upon perceiving John's discomfort, she feels uncomfortable herself. Previously Marci was cozy, and after watching John, she may not physically feel cold, but she does have a sense of distress, of waiting something to change so that she might feel better. Empathy on Marci's part also means that she has a sense of relief when the window is finally closed, even if she does not physically feel warmer. When Hume uses the word "sympathy," might he mean something closer to the contemporary connotation of the word "empathy"? An examination of Hume's own words bears out this possibility:

No quality of human nature is more remarkable, both in itself and its consequences, than the propensity we have to sympathize with others, and to receive by communication their inclinations and sentiments, however different from, or even contrary to, our own. (Hume 1948, 4–5)

We may begin with considering anew the nature and force of *sympathy*. The minds of all men are similar in their feelings and operations; nor can any one be actuated by any affection of which all others are not in the same degree susceptible. As in strings equally wound up the motion of one communicates itself to the rest, so all the affections readily pass from one person to another, and beget correspondent movements in every human creature. When I see the effects of passion in the voice and gesture of any person, my mind immediately passes from these effects to their causes, and forms such a lively idea of the passion as is presently converted into the passion itself. (Hume 1948, 132)

Stueber concurs, echoing that "... in Hume the concept of sympathy shows a multidimensionality similar to that of the concept of empathy in social psychology" (Stueber 2006, 29). Hume cannot recover his moral theory for the autistic moral agent by claiming that sympathy and empathy are distinct concepts—it is clear that Hume means by "sympathy" what is meant today by "empathy." Another means to recover the Humean moral theory needs to be employed.

Kennett does not conclude that persons with autism are outside the moral realm, or are beyond moral agency, thereby rejecting the second strategy. She locates several anecdotal examples of autistic individuals who do possess a moral sense, and in some cases, a strong sense of justice or fairness. Kennett's claims are in keeping with Blair's and Grant et al.'s empirical findings that persons with autism do recognize moral questions. If empirical evidence gives us reasons for thinking that persons with autism can recognize moral questions, and thus fulfill this necessary condition to act as moral agents, then the proper response is not to reject the autistic person as moral agent, but rather, to dismiss Humean moral theory.

Thus, the third response—to find an alternative conception of morality that accommodates the autistic moral agent—must be pursued. Kennett believes that Kant's moral theory will accommodate the autistic moral agent.

Kennett's Cautious Embrace and
Benn's Rejection of Kantian Theories

Kennett believes that "a clear advantage of a Kantian account of moral reasoning and moral motivation is that it grants full moral agency to morally conscientious autistic people . . ." (Kennett 2002, 355). There are places in Kant's discussion of morality in which he states that feelings such as empathy are not necessary, or even helpful, for an agent to perform morally worthy action. Kant believes that feelings do not shape moral duty, and in fact feelings can lead us astray from what moral duty requires of us. On this point, Kant's moral theory would appear to be quite attractive for autistic moral agents. Yet other elements of Kant's moral theory may ultimately be impractical for the person who lacks a theory of mind. Both the strengths and the weaknesses of Kant's moral theory merit consideration.

Supporters of Kantian moral theory as applicable for autistic moral agents might turn to the First Section of the *Groundwork*, in which Kant presents his Three Propositions of Morality. The First Proposition is that an action has moral worth only when it is done from duty. While discussing the first Proposition, Kant considers the relationship between emotions and our moral duties. He presents three necessary conditions for an act to be done from duty: (1) the act must be "in accord" with duty, (2) the agent who performs the action must recognize that this action is what duty requires, and (3) the agent must action from the recognition that this act is what duty requires (Kant 1956). Thus, an action is morally worthy when it is performed out of the correct motivation—the recognition that this action is the one that duty requires—rather than out of an inclination, out of love, or other sentiments. In keeping with the dismissal of inclination as a causal contributor to morally worthy action, Kant rejects sympathy as a motivation:

> To help others where one can is a duty, and besides this there are
> many spirits of so sympathetic a temper that, without any further
> motive of vanity or self-interest, they find an inner pleasure in spread-
> ing happiness around them and can take delight in the contentment
> of others as their own work. Yet I maintain that in such a case an

action of this kind, however right and however amiable it may be, has still no genuinely moral worth.

. . . Suppose then that the mind of this friend of man were over-clouded by sorrows of his own which extinguished all sympathy with the fate of others, but that he still had power to help those in distress, though no longer stirred by the need of others because sufficiently occupied with his own; and suppose that, when no longer moved by any inclination, he tears himself out of this deadly insensibility and does the action without any inclination for the sake of duty alone; then for the first time his action has its genuine moral worth. (Kant 1956, 66)

Kant recognizes that emotion can make us receptive to the concept of duty, but it is not a necessary condition for an act to be done from duty, and in fact it can mislead us. The agent who acts in accord with duty, not because of the recognition that this action is what duty requires, but out of inclination, sympathy, empathy, or "pathological love" does not act morally, for this agent's actions are changeable and contingent on a feeling that cannot be the basis for a universal and necessary morality. These emotions may result in an agent acting in such a way that is in accord with what duty requires—they can serve as a motivation for an agent to act in a way that is consistent with her duty—but they do not serve a role in the supreme principle of all duty.

From this perspective, Kant's theory may prove more attractive than Hume's for autistic individuals. Hume's theory relies on feelings of empathy which are problematic for autistic persons. Perhaps the autistic person will be more inclined to take a Kantian perspective, as it is more rule-governed, and relies less on sympathy and other emotions (Kennett 2002, 351). As long as an agent recognizes that duty requires a particular course of action, and that the agent acts in keeping with this recognition, then the agent has performed a morally worthy action. Kennett states, "Kant's point in stripping away sympathy as a motive in his examples in the *Groundwork* is to reveal the essence of moral agency, the concern to act in accordance with reason which animates agency and which we cannot do without" (Kennett 2002, 355). The autistic agent employs a "cold methodology" of intellect without emotion or motivation, as opposed to a "hot methodology" which involves simulation of others' mental states (Kennett 2002, 352). Kantian moral theory's eschewing of emotions, such as sympathy, might make Kantian moral theory more attractive to the autistic moral agent.[7]

Kennett's full embrace of a Kantian moral theory is tempered by her recognition of the limits autism can place on a person's understanding of the self. Without an understanding of one's own conscious states, motivations, and intentions, *per* Frith and Happé, for example, moral agency would be compromised. If this is the case, then even the cold methodology of Kant may not be sufficient to present a practicable moral theory for autistic individuals.[8]

While a cold methodology advocated by Kant initially seems more appealing than the hot methodology advocated by Hume, there are two reasons why employing Kantian moral theory is more elusive for autistic persons than it would first appear. The first is that the role of emotions is not as clear in Kantian theory as it would appear from the above passages in the *Groundwork*. While Kennett may be correct in dismissing a Humean moral theory for relying too much on feelings of sympathy to be workable for the autistic agent, in *The Doctrine of Virtue* Kant observes that cultivating sympathy can contribute to the performance of duty in some cases. Sympathy can be of some value in the Kantian system, although Kant grants that it can also lead us astray. Kennett quotes Kant that without "moral feeling" an individual would be "morally dead" (Kennett 2002, 353). Feelings—even feelings of sympathy—can have a role in Kantian moral theory.

A second reason for rejecting a Kantian moral theory's feasibility for autistic individuals is that some formulations of the categorical imperative may not be workable for individuals who lack theory of mind. Kant believes that there is a single supreme principle of all duty, the categorical imperative, and he presents several extensionally equivalent formulations of that single imperative. Two formulations are particularly difficult for autistic individuals.

Kant urges us to "Act on the maxims of a member who makes universal laws for a merely possible kingdom of ends" (Kant 1956, 106). This formulation is effectively a social contract among all members of moral society. According to Kant, human beings, in virtue of their rationality, are the sources of the moral law: "the Idea of the will of every rational being as a will which makes universal law" (Kant 1956,

98). The social contract stipulates that all persons are lawgivers in a society in which each person is the source of the moral law. Of course not everyone recognizes this, and does not always act in accordance with this notion. The kingdom of ends—the kingdom of rational persons who create the moral law and recognize the source of the moral law in others—is thus a merely possible place. When acting in accordance with our moral duty, however, we act in keeping with the recognition of such a kingdom of ends.

Benn believes that social contact theories, including Kant-influenced social contract theories, are not workable for the autistic agent. Social contract theories require some level of reciprocity among agents. The kingdom of ends formulation of the categorical imperative requires each person to recognize certain facts about other persons, and to act in keeping with this recognition. However, Benn believes that autistic individuals are incapable of exercising this reciprocity, and thus are left out of any social contract:

> The guiding thought here is that morality is that set of principles that rational agents could freely agree to observe, on condition that everyone else observe them as well. And commitment to such an agreement entails a commitment to reciprocity. If certain individuals are incapable of understanding the need for reciprocity, or of entertaining the moral feelings that normally motivate its observance, then for that reason they exclude themselves from the agreement, and may be treated in ways in which normal people may never treat one another. (Benn 1999, 38)

Benn claims that social contract theories cannot be successfully employed by autistic agents. It is important to recognize that the kind of reciprocity that Benn cites here is emotional reciprocity. Nussbaum also discusses the limits of Kantian social contracts for some persons with disabilities, but dismisses them based on a different sense of reciprocity. According to Nussbaum, Kant would disqualify "passive citizens" who are "underlings of the commonwealth," any individual who "cannot support himself by his own industry" from entering into a social contract (Nussbaum 2006, 52). Thus, Kant does not conceive of severely disabled persons as members of the social contract. However, Benn's argument is not about dependency—which is fortunate, since

Nussbaum correctly observes that some high-functioning persons with autism or Asperger's may well carry out lives that are not marked by dependency on others. Rather, it is an argument about the possibility of even entering into a social contract when an autistic person's conception of others is limited.

Benn's position, as argued in chapter 2, is controversial. Benn's conclusions about the elimination of autistic individuals from the moral community were rejected earlier. It is possible to grant Benn his point about the inapplicability of social contract theories for autistic agents, while not buying wholesale into his rejection of autistic persons from the moral community. The kingdom of ends formulation may be salvageable, however. Another formulation of the categorical imperative, the formulation of the principle of autonomy, is closely connected to the formulation based on a kingdom of ends. One formulation of the principle of autonomy might read, "So act that your will can regard itself at the same time as making universal law through its maxims" (Aune 1979, 112). On Kant's account, individuals who recognize that they make the moral law through their own maxims and conform to the moral law by virtue of this fact are autonomous. Kennett asserts that the autistic person is "not morally autonomous" (Kennett 2002, 351), and thus may provide an additional objection to the use of Kantian ethics for autistic persons. Kennett invokes Velleman's definition of autonomy, "the inclination towards conscious control, towards behaving 'in, and out of, a knowledge of what you're doing'" (Kennett 2002, 353). This notion of autonomy stresses authenticity; in contrast, the Kantian notion of autonomy consists in being the author of universal law and acting, not from inclination but, from that law. Kennett says that while most persons with autism do not have moral autonomy, high-functioning individuals, such as some with Asperger's, "can achieve moral autonomy by other means [rather than simulation theory]. It appears that they can develop or discover moral rules and principles of conduct for themselves by reasoning, as they would in other matters, on the basis of patient explicit inquiry, reliance on testimony and inference from past situations" (Kennett 2002, 351). In other words, some people with autism do have the requisite moral autonomy. But it is unclear whether Kennett and Kant are considering an identical notion of "autonomy." If there is an equivocation, this would undermine the applicability of the formulation of the principle of autonomy for autistic persons, even very high-functioning autistic persons. In summary, the kingdom of ends formulation was rejected on the basis of Benn's observations about the inability of autistic persons to enter into the right form of reciprocity necessary for social contracts; the principle of autonomy formulation was rejected on the basis of the fact that the autonomy necessary for this formulation may not be possessed by autistic agents.

Another, yet more problematic formulation of the categorical imperative, states "Act in such a way that you always treat humanity, whether in your own person or in the person of any other, never simply as a means, but always at the same time as an end" (Kant 1956, 96). Kant believes the supreme principle of all morality must take into consideration the fact that human beings are objective ends with dignity and value in themselves, rather than mere subjective ends. Subjective ends can be used by others and then be thrown away, whereas objective ends, having value in themselves, must be treated with respect. Human beings have intrinsic value, not merely instrumental or extrinsic value. Thus, no human can be treated "merely as a means," but must instead be treated as an end in him or herself. What, though, does it mean to treat others as ends in themselves, and not merely as means? Treating others as ends in themselves may require us to realize and share others' ends, and to act in a positive fashion so as to further those ends (Aune 1979, 78). Agents who are ends in themselves "are regarded as 'persons' rather than as 'things' because they are by nature free and rational, able and obligated to set goals, to recognize the existence of objective ends, to make genuine choices, and to enact and act on genuinely universal laws of conduct for themselves and all others" (Sullivan 1989, 197).

Can the autistic individual treat others as ends in themselves, rather than merely as means to some other end? It is questionable whether a person whose ability to ascribe intentionality to others is compromised is able to conceive of persons as objective ends. Treating another person as an end in him- or herself implies recognizing others as having intentional attitudes distinct from your own, such that you do not merely use this other person as an extension of your own will, but as an individual whose life projects demand consideration. On the unified consciousness view, however, autistic people may be unable to ascribe intentional attitudes distinct from their own. A result of this failure, as mentioned earlier, is the failure of ST as a method of explaining human actions by autistic persons. Thus, this formulation of the categorical imperative is also problematic for the autistic individual.[9]

There is a lack of fit between Kantian moral theory and the autistic moral agent. Benn does not claim that the inapplicability of Kantian moral theory for autistic agents is a reason for rejecting a Kantian theory; rather, insofar as some autistic individuals are incapable of feeling reciprocity, we may be permitted to treat them in ways that we could not morally permissibly treat others. Even if Benn is mistaken, the formulation of the categorical imperative that states that we should not treat others merely as a means presents its own difficulties for autistic agency. However, the tension between Kantian morality and autistic moral agents can be resolved in another way: the fact that a Kantian moral theory cannot accommodate the autistic individual may be reason for rejecting Kantian theory, not for excluding the autistic person. New approaches to moral theory are required.

Particularism and an Ethic of *Prima Facie* Duties

Moral particularism holds that an act token's normative status is determined independently of moral principles, whereas an ethic of *prima facie* duties holds that the moral status of act tokens is determined by reference to competing principles. The two would seem to have little in common, and are in fact often juxtaposed as embodying two extreme positions in ethical theory—the former eschews all moral rules or principles, whereas the later embraces rules or principles. One trait they do share is that both are unworkable for autistic moral agents.

Moral particularism was borne of ethical theory's discontents. Particularists find ethical principles too constrictive and too inflexible. Ethical principles fail to acknowledge that what can seem to be a reason to do something in one case can in fact be a reason *not* to do that same thing in a similar case. The fact that a job applicant *will vastly enjoy his work* might count in favor of hiring that applicant; the fact that the applicant for the job of executioner *will vastly enjoy his work* counts in favor of hiring someone else—"the behavior of a reason (or of a consideration that serves as a reason) in a new case cannot be predicted from its behavior elsewhere" (Dancy 1993, 60). Rather than practice a moral generalism or universalizability that relies on often wrong abstract principles, particularists look instead to a holism of reasons for performing one action rather than another. These reasons cannot be cashed out as moral rules or principles because rules or principles fail to consider the situational complexity of morality. This approach is thought to be more pluralistic than traditional moral theory, which is hamstrung by its abstract principles. According to the particularist, the "salient features" of a case determine which action is morally right or wrong, rather than general principles. Particularists embrace "coherence in a moral outlook" (Dancy 1993, 63).

The autistic individual may have difficulty following particularism. One of these difficulties may stem from the properties that a moral agent would need to have in order to be a successful particularist. Jonathan Dancy writes:

> To be so consistently successful, we need to have a broad range of sensitivities, so that no relevant feature escapes us, and we do not mistake its relevance either. But that is all there is to say on this matter. To have the relevant sensitivities just is to be able to get things right case by case. The only remaining question is how we might get into this enviable state. And the answer is that for us it is probably too late. As Aristotle held, moral education is the key; for those who are past educating, there is no real remedy. (Dancy 1993, 64)

According to Dancy, any person so far gone that she is reading his book is beyond moral education, but presumably there are a few impressionable youths who still stand a chance. Moral education must start early. The question for the autistic person is not, "Is it too late to begin moral education?" but "Was it not always too late?" Has the autistic agent always lacked the "broad range of sensitivities" needed to be a successful particularist? Lawrence Blum observes that "situational perception, judgment, and particularistic sensitivities are as central to [moral] agency as is commitment to principle" (Blum 1988, 723). These capacities may be the very ones that are too daunting for the autistic individual. Jay Garfield observes that for two moral agents to see the same properties as salient those agents "must, in the existential sense, inhabit the same world; we must, at a fundamental level, care about the same things" (Garfield 2000, 203). It seems contrary to the spirit of particularism to posit a set of principles that would demonstrate whether two individuals inhabited the same world, or cared about the same things. But being an agent with intentions and having your distinct intentions recognized would seem to be, at the most basic level, necessary for two individuals to occupy that same world, and to care about the same things. The discussion here parallels earlier discussion about the failure of simulation. The failure of the autistic person to care about what others care about—the failure of empathy required for true simulation—undermined Humean moral theory's applicability for the autistic individual. Given Garfield's claim about mutual caring as necessary for agents to recognize salience, it would appear that the same lessons apply to particularism.

A second, but related, difficulty for particularism's applicability to autistic moral agents is the situational aspect which disdains rules in favor of a more holistic approach to ethics. This approach seems to be one that would be daunting for persons with autism given the hypotheses that symptoms of autism are manifestations of weak central coherence (O'Loughlin and Thagard 2000; Happé 2000). Perhaps for this reason a more rule-governed approach to ethics is called for. Thus an ethic of *prima facie* duties now merits consideration.

The theory forwarded by Tom Beauchamp and James Childress in their influential *Principles of Biomedical Ethics* is an example of an ethic of *prima facie* duties, as are the guidelines set forward in the *Belmont Report* (Beauchamp and Childress 2001; National Commission for the Protection of Human Subjects of Biomedical and Behavioral Research 1978). While both the *Belmont Report* and Beauchamp and Childress's work have their detractors (Ainslie 2002; Buchanan et al. 2000; Gert et al. 1997), the impact of both in contemporary bioethics is unquestionable. An ethic of *prima facie* duties is one that postulates that there are competing moral duties or principles that confront agents, the stringency of which must be ascertained in order to determine the overriding moral duty or obligation in each situation. None of these duties or principles is absolute; their relative weight can change with changing circumstances. In some cases it might be acceptable to lie in order to spare someone's feelings, but in other cases it might be imperative to tell the truth even if others will be hurt in the process. W. D. Ross postulated seven *prima facie* duties: duties of fidelity, which include truth-telling and promise-keeping; duties of reparation; duties of gratitude; duties of justice; duties of beneficence; duties of self-improvement; and duties of nonmaleficence (Ross 2002). When a moral question arises an agent must first consider which of the *prima facie* duties is applicable to the circumstances, and then determine which of the applicable duties is most stringent in the particular case. For example, an agent might recognize the duty of fidelity in not keeping a secret from a close friend, but she might also recognize a duty of beneficence toward that friend in playing along in the planning of his surprise birthday party. Ross believed that all humans share similar moral intuitions, which allow them both to determine what the *prima facie* duties actually are, as well as determine their relative stringency in a particular case. Ross often refers to that which is "self-evident," "what we think," "reflect on" or "apprehend" as intuitively known claims, which belie any attempts at further rigor or systematization:

> . . . we see the *prima facie* rightness of an act which would be the fulfilment of a particular promise, and of another which would be the fulfilment of another promise, and when we have reached sufficient maturity to think in general terms, we apprehend *prima facie* rightness to belong to the nature of any fulfilment of promise. What comes first in time is the apprehension of the self-evident *prima facie* rightness of an individual act of a particular type. From this we come by reflection to apprehend the self-evident general principle of *prima facie* duty. (Ross 2002, 33)
> The existing body of moral convictions of the best people is the cumulative product of the moral reflection of many generations, which has developed an extremely delicate power of appreciation of moral distinctions; and this the theorist cannot afford to treat with anything other than the greatest respect. (Ross 2002, 41)

> For the estimation of the comparative stringency of these *prima facie*
> obligations no general rules can, so far as I can see, be laid down. . . .
> This sense of our particular duty in particular circumstances, pre-
> ceded and informed by the fullest reflection we can bestow on the act
> in all its bearings, is highly fallible, but it is the only guide we have to
> our duty. (Ross 2002, 41–42)

Beauchamp and Childress offer their own version of an ethic of
prima facie duties in which they postulate four principles of biomedical
ethics: autonomy, nonmaleficence, beneficence, and justice. Beauchamp
and Childress claim that their four principles "do not constitute a general
moral theory," and rather "provide only a framework for identifying and
reflecting on moral problems" (Beauchamp and Childress 2001, 15).
However it is worth considering how they believe that conflicts among
prima facie principles should be resolved. Beauchamp and Childress
caution that even if rules exist that will delineate the more stringent obligations, "in light of the enormous range of possibilities for contingent
conflicts among rules, even the firmest rules are better construed as
evolving rather than finished products" (Beauchamp and Childress 2001,
19). They recommend guidelines that can be employed so that the balancing of competing principles is not merely intuitive or subjective. But
even with these guidelines, they conclude their discussion by observing
that "Honesty about the process of balancing and overriding compels us
to return to our early discussion of dilemmas and to acknowledge that in
some circumstances we will not be able to determine which moral norm
is overriding" (Beauchamp and Childress 2001, 21).

A challenge an ethic of *prima facie* duties poses for the autistic individual emerges at the second step—arbitrating amongst competing
duties. As observed by John Lawson, the autistic individual may find
it particularly difficult to weigh competing *prima facie* duties (Lawson 2003). Lawson does not dispute the theory of mind thesis, but
believes that the theory of mind thesis is a subset of a larger thesis, the
Depth Accessibility Difficulty (DAD) model. The DAD model proposes that persons with autism spectrum conditions reduce the world
"to closed systems of atomistic (essentially unconnected) actualities,
with process of change reduced in effect to differences" (Lawson 2003,
197). Persons with DAD have difficulty dealing with deep structures,

internal relations, open systems, and highly interconnected phenomena. Lawson forwards the DAD model as a way of embracing four seemingly distinct theories of autism: the theory of mind thesis, the systematizing-empathizing thesis, the weak central coherence thesis, and the weak executive function thesis. Lawson contends that the first two do a fine job explaining some of the social deficits faced by persons with autism; the latter two succeed in explaining other, more mechanistic processing deficits, as well as certain strengths that some autistic persons demonstrate with respect to folk physics and sorting tasks. The DAD model, in his estimation, brings together the strengths of all of these theories, as each theory can be understood as a subset of the DAD model. Lawson considers several consequences of the DAD thesis, including its implications for conversational pragmatics and moral theory:

> ... people with [autism spectrum conditions] are likely to have difficulties in dealing with any outcomes that are determined by multiple factors, i.e., which have many and changing causes.... For example, with respect to moral codes, it may be good to tell the truth but at times it may be better to keep a secret (e.g. about a birthday party or a friend's rule breaking behaviour). Sometimes it is good to join in a conversation, at other times it is more polite not to do so. (Lawson 2003, 200)

Lawson perceives that the person with depth accessibility difficulties would be unable to arbitrate among competing *prima facie* duties. On one hand, there is the obligation that one does not keep secrets; but on the other hand, the party will not be as fun if the guest of honor knows what is being planned. Knowing which of the competing *prima facie* duties is more stringent—the duty of fidelity or the duty of beneficence—would be difficult for the autistic person on the DAD model. Lawrence Blum, in his criticism of an ethic of *prima facie* duties, cites this as a failure of "moral perception"—the inability of an agent when examining alternative actions to "perceive their moral character accurately" (Blum 1991, 84). Thus, the second step that an agent must undertake when using an ethic of *prima facie* duties—arbitrating among competing duties to determine which is correct—would be beyond the capabilities of some autistic agents.

Less obvious problems for an ethic of *prima facie* duties emerge at the first step—the point at which an agent first recognizes that a given *prima facie* duty even exists. Given Ross's observation above, the initial recognition of moral duties such as fidelity or beneficence requires the same type of moves that might challenge the person who is impaired by DAD. But there is a second reason the recognition of *prima facie* duties might elude the person with autism. Ross's view is that *prima facie* duties grow out of special types of relationships that we enter into which serve as the basis for moral obligations, such as "promisee to promiser, of creditor to debtor, of wife to husband, of child to parent, of friend to friend, of fellow countryman to fellow countryman, and the like; and each of these relations is the foundation of a *prima facie* duty, which is more or less incumbent upon me according to the circumstances of the case" (Ross 2002, 19). Given the difficulties that persons with autism have entering into relationships, or recognizing the complexities of human relationships, it is possible that the moral obligations that emerge in virtue of these relationships would escape the person with autism. If the complexities of certain relationships remain a mystery, then the moral obligations that emerge from those relationships may also remain a mystery. Thus, even the first step—recognizing the relevant *prima facie* duties in a particular situation—could stymie autistic moral agents. For these reasons, an ethic of *prima facie* duties does not appear workable for the autistic individual.

In summary, several different moral theories have been presented, each of which may be problematic for the individual with autism. What are the practical consequences if some moral theories cannot be used by both autistic and non-autistic individuals alike? The following discussion illustrates the way in which a gulf between applicable moral theories has practical implications.

A Problem Raised by Incompatible Moral Theories: Should Adults with Autism be "Cured"?

If I could snap my fingers and be nonautistic, I would not—because then I wouldn't be me. Autism is part of who I am.

TEMPLE GRANDIN, AS QUOTED BY OLIVER SACKS (SACKS 1995, 291)

Imagine this scenario: a "cure" for autism is found which can be given to adults with autism. Persons who have lived for years without theory of mind are administered this cure, and for the first time are able to effortlessly ascribe intentionality to others. Inability to employ the pragmatics of language and impaired empathy are left behind as persons with autism enter the world of non-autistic individuals. Should the cure be given to adults with autism? The immediate response might be "yes"—surely any condition that can be cured should be cured. Chapters 2 and 3 illustrate why this is a more complex question than it would first appear.

One reason to question a cure concerns the pain that can result from a fully functioning theory of mind. Much of the discussion in chapter 2 considered the goods that accrue from relationships with other persons and the objective value of relationships. But just as there are some goods that we can only obtain with theory of mind, so too there are some evils that are bad in part because of the recognition of having these ills visited upon the victim. Parfit's objective list of bad states of affairs, including being betrayed, manipulated, slandered, and deceived is only possible for the individual with a functional theory of mind. Each of these states of affairs is possible only when an agent is aware than other agents hold a particular set of beliefs about him. It is meaningless to claim to be betrayed or deceived by someone, or something, that lacks intentionality. The person who lacks a theory of mind is blissfully ignorant of being ridiculed or lied to. There are many bad things that cannot happen to the person who lacks theory of mind. Some might argue that those ills are better off avoided.

There are two possible objections to this claim. The first is to claim that just because an agent does not *know* that he is being betrayed does not mean that he *has not* been betrayed; the badness of being betrayed compromises the goodness of an agent's life, even if that agent is never aware of the betrayal. Thus, even those who lack theory of mind are harmed by the bad states of affairs that would appear to accrue only to individuals who did have theory of mind. A response to this claim is that it does not say enough about the reciprocal nature of human interaction. If a betrayal is just as bad even if you do not know that it is happening, is being loved just as good if you do not know that it is happening either? What about the agent who goes through life unaware that it is even possible to be loved, because he fails to recognize agency in others? If the goods in life like being loved and trusted, are muted by a failure of theory of mind, then so too are the ills in life muted. The objection still stands, but it is weakened somewhat by the reply that both the goods, and the ills, of human life are dampened when an agent fails to have a fully functional theory of mind.

A second objection is that while the harms of deceit or betrayal are real, the good in being able to bear positive reciprocal attitudes outweighs those harms. Thus, the formerly autistic individual benefits, on balance, by having a functional theory of mind, even if some harms result from possessing theory of mind. Additionally, the good of those surrounded by autistic persons, such as their families, may be best served by bringing the autistic person into the world shared by non-autistic persons. This argument is decidedly act-utilitarian: the reasoning is about trade-offs between the good and the harm that accrues from having theory of mind, both for the person whose theory of mind is in question, and for those affected by that person's acquisition of theory of mind. As with any act-utilitarian claim, though, it is not the case that a given type of act will always be morally right or morally wrong. Rather, a case-by-case assessment of the utilities involved must be considered. Furthermore, as discussed earlier in this chapter, utilitarianism may lack much of its appeal for persons with autism, as Mill's "ultimate sanction of utility" is not persuasive to the person with autism. Thus, this objection may work in some, but not in all cases, and even in those cases in which non-autistic persons are convinced, autistic persons may be less so.

Some people may argue that to deprive any autistic person of a fully functioning theory of mind is to fail to recognize the kind of thing that humans are. In keeping with Nussbaum, there are certain capacities all humans share. To deny any human the ability to act in keeping with those capacities is to do harm to him *qua human*. Yes, it is true that there will be pain that will result from conferring a theory of mind on a person who previously did not have a fully functioning theory of mind, but to knowingly keep theory of mind from an individual who lacks it is to deny that individual's humanity. The argument here is not an argument from costs and benefits, as proponents of this argument must concede that to give a person who previously had no theory of mind the ability to easily and effortlessly ascribe intentionality to others may do more harm than good in a small number of cases. This argument is one that urges a bridging of the gap between the autistic and non-autistic person, but unapologetically says that we should bridge the gap only by bringing the autistic person over to the non-autistic side. Perhaps after that we should just burn the bridge—why would anyone ever want to go back?

This leads to the second reason to resist moving the autistic person into the world of the non-autistic: perhaps the rules governing the two worlds may be so different that reasons non-autistic persons cite for moving the autistic person into their world may simply not apply to the autistic person. As discussed in this chapter, the unique deficits faced by autistic persons make some of the most prominent moral theories inapplicable to the autistic person. When the moral question "Should this person be cured of autism?" is asked, whose morality should govern the answer?[10] If act-utilitarianism does not give us a hard-and-fast answer, and is not persuasive to the autistic person anyway, then what are we left with? Humean, Kantian, Rossian, and particularist moral theories are not applicable to one of the parties in question. So which moral theory *should* guide the answer? How can two populations arbitrate among competing, non-extensionally equivalent, moral theories? This problem has been cited as a reason to reject subjectivism and other types of relativism. It has been cited as a reason to reject a feminist or feminine ethic, which would argue that men and women do not merely speak of moral problems in a different voice, but are governed by competing, and incompatible, moral theories. Theory of mind deficits, however, seem to speak to a much more profound gulf between persons than either gender or culture. As considered in chapter 2, these deficits address significant aspects of what it means to be a member of the moral community, or to lead a good human life. The possibility of a person who was cut off in a fundamental way from other persons might have been considered previously as a thought experiment to test the boundaries of different moral claims. Persons with autism make that thought experiment a reality.

The point in raising the moral questions surrounding a cure is to illustrate the uniquely confounding problems confronting ethics and autism. No one who studies ethics is under any illusions that there are easy answers to questions in metaethics, normative ethics, or applied ethics. But the autistic individual, in virtue of his unique attributes, presents exceptional challenges to those who would answer ethical questions. The problem of a cure—as far off as that might be—is only one bioethical question that emerges when considering persons with autism. Two other problems concern the use of genetic technologies to prevent the birth of persons with autism, and the use of persons with autism in research studies. These questions are the subjects of the next two chapters.

Voices of Autism

Donna Williams's *autobiographical writings include many of the same themes as those addressed by Wendy Lawson and Gunilla Gerland. Williams's first book,* Nobody Nowhere, *begins with her childhood and school years during which time she experienced sensory difficulties and alienation from other children. She was unable to abide high-pitched sounds or human touch; bright lights were by turns "intolerable or mesmerizing" (Williams 1992, 207). Her parents' contentious relationship exacerbated her problems. She left home when she was a teenager, and like Gerland was involved in a series of failed relationships. Williams found "whole people" difficult to understand, especially nuanced aspects of reciprocal relationships (William 1992, 35). She moved from relationship to relationship, job to job, home to home—and in some cases home to homelessness—never knowing the source of her estrangement from others.*

Williams concocted a pair of façades, Carol and Willie, that she hid behind in order to navigate the social world. These façades were the means by which she communicated to those in the outside world, an attempt to break free of the insular world of autism (Williams 1992, 138). Carol was the socially engaging one, but was also prone to be too agreeable, leading Donna into bad relationships. Willie was competent in employment situations, but occasionally disagreeable. Only in her early twenties was Donna diagnosed with autism, a revelation that finally enabled her to make sense of a lifetime of sensory overload and social isolation.

Somebody Somewhere, Williams's second book, chronicles the period of time immediately after the publication of Nobody Nowhere. *Armed with an understanding of autism, Donna is able to slowly shake off Carol* and Willie, and take steps to engage "the world" as opposed to living in what she calls "my world." With the publication of Nobody Nowhere Donna discovered autistic children and adults all over the world.

At the conclusion of Somebody Somewhere Williams stresses that persons with autism cannot simply be taught to experience certain thoughts or feelings, or be made to feel emotionally for others. A person with autism can learn what he or she is supposed to feel in a particular situation, and then act in keeping with those feelings, "but that doesn't make it your own, and an idea is never a feeling, just a memory or a stored mental repertoire of how one appears" (Williams 1994, 214). Williams closes with the assertion that "autism is not me," and instead is that which "tries to rob me of a life, of friendship, of caring, of sharing, of using my intelligence, of being affected . . . it tries to bury me alive" (Williams 1994, 238).

4

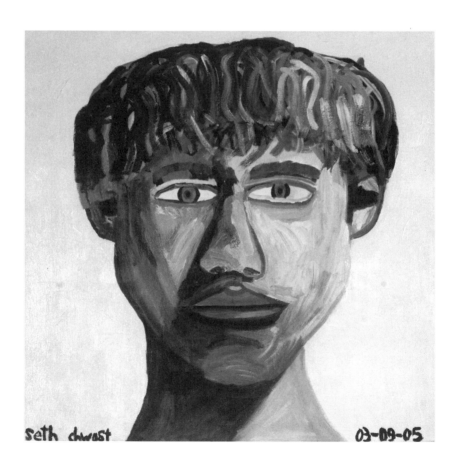

SETH CHWAST, *SELF-STUDY #3, SMALL SELF-STUDY IN BLACK AND WHITE*

Autism and Genetic Technologies

Current estimates are that between 30 and 50 percent of cases of autism are inherited genetically, although few cases overall are directly inherited because people with autism rarely have children (Siegel 1996; Frith 2003). Evidence also exists for a genetic basis for some cases of Asperger's syndrome (Ghaziuddin 2005). Rett Syndrome, a rare condition which is believed to fall on the autism spectrum, is the result of a mutation in the MECP2 gene (Wade 2007). Researchers have located genes that may result in greater vulnerability to environmental triggers that may contribute to autism, creating the possibility that genetic factors and environmental factors combine to create susceptibility to autism (Campbell et al. 2006). Between 30 and 40 percent of autism cases appear to have no genetic component, and instead may be the result of birth- or pregnancy-related causes (Baron-Cohen and Bolton 1993). Some researchers claim that it is not autism per se that is inherited, but rather a range of psychological difficulties which subsequently result in autism (Baron-Cohen and Bolton 1993). For example, approximately 10 percent of autism cases are a result of Fragile X syndrome, a congenital condition. Other studies point to a genetic basis for either abnormal brain development or faulty serotonin processing (Kuehn 2006). Even in the cases in which autism is the result of another condition that has a genetic component, questions about the use of genetic technologies and autism persist. The fact that a significant number of autism cases *do* have a genetic basis raises questions about what we can or should do with emerging genetic technologies that have an impact on the autistic population.

Today we have no knowledge of an "autism gene," akin to a gene for Huntington's disease, although certain chromosomal regions have been located which are implicated in autism (Monastersky 2007; Autism Genome Project Consortium 2007). Nor do we know which set of genes might indicate a likelihood of developing autistic symptoms, akin to genes such as BRCA1 or BRCA2, which increase the likelihood that a woman will develop breast or ovarian cancer. Perhaps there are genetic factors that make some individuals more vulnerable to environmental factors, the combination of which results in autism. Even if an "autism gene" were located, there is no guarantee that the initially discovered gene would allow us to draw distinctions among those who are most or least affected by the disorder (Frith 2003). There is evidence that "mild degrees of mindblindness" on the part of parents may be one aspect of a broader condition (Baron-Cohen 2000a). However, the fact that a significant percentage of cases of autism are attributable to genetic factors leads to hard ethical questions. Most of what we know about the genetics of autism will not confront us with these questions today. But the future will bring us closer to difficult choices about genetics and autism.[1] One of the most difficult is whether parents should use genetic technologies to prevent the birth of children with autism.

One answer to this question, as simple as it is controversial, is to perform a straightforward cost-benefit analysis. There is a great deal of talk about an epidemic of autism, and while there is a dispute as to whether the *actual* numbers of autistic persons are increasing, or whether it is only the numbers of persons *diagnosed* with autism that has increased, the increases themselves are not in dispute. The number of persons diagnosed with autism has increased from 22,664 in the United States ten years ago to over 141,022 in 2005 (Gross 2005). The current estimate is that one in one hundred fifty children in the United States develop autism or an autism spectrum disorder such as Asperger's by the age of eight (Carey 2007). Explanations vary from environmental factors, which may or may not be interacting with genetic predispositions toward autism, to revised diagnostic criteria which result in more persons being diagnosed with autism than in the past, to the possibility that greater public awareness has increased the likelihood that one will receive this diagnosis. For example, one oft-quoted study observes that the number of children diagnosed with autism in California increased from 5.78 children in ten thousand in 1987 to 14.89 in ten thousand by 1994 (Croen et al. 2002). However, this increase was accompanied by a decrease in the number of children diagnosed with mental retardation, a decrease that nearly mirrored the increase in the number of children diagnosed with autism (Frith 2003). Paul Shattuck found similar figures: from 1994 until 2003 the prevalence of autism rose from 0.6 to 3.1 per one thousand in the United States, even as the rate of mental retardation fell by 2.8 per one thousand (Shattuck 2006). These numbers could be explained by many factors; in addition to those mentioned above (e.g., greater public awareness of autism, more precise diagnostic assessments), it may be that a diagnosis of "autism" is less socially stigmatizing and thus more often applied than "mental retardation."[2] One much-disputed theory is that childhood vaccines containing mercury cause an increase in the number of children with autism, although this theory has been largely discredited (Harris 2005; Harris and O'Connor 2005).

As the number of persons diagnosed with autism increases, the resources needed to appropriately care for and educate persons with autism increases. Estimates for the annual cost of education for a child with autism range from twenty-five thousand (Freudenheim 2004) to sixty thousand U.S. dollars (Carey 2004; Daly 2005). It is a mistake to deny that these cost-benefit issues exist, or to deny that they have been cited in the past as justification for using genetic technologies to prevent the birth of persons with certain conditions.[3] At the same time, there is a terrible history of eugenics in the United States, much of which was fostered by cost-benefit thinking, as well as notions of what it means for a person to be "unfit" or "feeble-minded." Cost-benefit thinking, in the form of what Allen Buchanan et al. call the "Public Health Model," was cited in the past as a justification for forced sterilizations and other unjust eugenic policies. This type of cost-benefit thinking is not a solution to questions about genetics and autism (Buchanan et al. 2000), because it sacrifices parental autonomy as well as justice to future persons.[4] As shown at the close of chapter 2, it is also a moral mistake to dismiss the autistic person from the moral community, assigning him to the realm of the "unfit" or "feeble-minded." Martha Nussbaum says that her theory of human capabilities would allow for genetic intervention in the case of severe cerebral palsy, but not in the case of Asperger's syndrome, because "there is a realistic prospect that they [persons with Asperger's] will attain the capabilities that we have evaluated as humanly central" (Nussbaum 2006, 193).[5] At the same time, Nussbaum does not rule out genetic interventions that would prevent the future birth of persons with Asperger's. A closer examination of arguments about genetics and autism is called for.

This chapter's first three sections each consider an argument against using genetic technologies to prevent the birth of children with autism: the parental autonomy argument, the social construction of disability argument, and an argument that draws an analogy between the Deaf community and communities of persons with autism. The strengths and weaknesses of each argument are considered, and each is ultimately rejected. After each of these arguments is discussed an argument based on the right to an open future, as well as objections to this argument, is presented. The chapter concludes with a discussion of a question that is closely related to the questions surrounding autism and genetics: given the significant ratio of boys to girls born with autism, is it permissible to use sex selection in an attempt to lower the likelihood that a child with autism will be born to at-risk families?

Parental Autonomy and a Failed Argument against Using Genetic Technologies

Some believe that it is the prerogative of parents to use—or not use—genetic technologies, even if the decision means that a child will be born with a condition such as autism. The argument proceeds from the claim that parents should have autonomy to do what they wish for their children, including their future children. Insofar as parents have autonomy rights with respect to choosing their children's schooling, choosing their children's healthcare, and choosing many other aspects of their children's lives, so too parents should have unchecked autonomy when it comes to employing, or failing to employ, genetic technologies. This position is consistent with what Buchanan et al. refer to as the "Personal Service Model"—genetic technologies should be used, or not used, on the basis of individuals' personal preferences (Buchanan et al. 2000). Thus, even if parents know that they can prevent a child from being born with autism, parental autonomy does not commit the parents to any course of action. The argument from parental autonomy can be represented in this way:

(1) Parents are permitted to exercise autonomy when making choices that affect their children's lives;

(2) If parents are permitted to exercise autonomy when making choices that affect their children's lives, then parents are permitted to exercise autonomy when making the choice as to whether their child is autistic;

(3) Therefore, parents are permitted to exercise autonomy when making the choice as to whether their child is autistic.

This argument is clearly unsound, as parents do not and should not have autonomy with respect to every aspect of their children's lives. There are some limits as to what it is permissible for parents to do when their actions affect their children's welfare, thereby casting doubt on the first premise of the argument. Buchanan et al. argue persuasively that just as there are limits on parental autonomy after a child is born, so too is it reasonable that limits are placed on parental autonomy prior to a child being born (Buchanan et al. 2000). No one, not even parents, should have unchecked autonomy when it comes to performing actions that may harm others. As argued in chapter 2, living an autistic life is not, *ceteris paribus,* as good a human life as that child's life had he not been born autistic. Thus, arguments from parental autonomy cannot be invoked to demonstrate that genetic technologies should not be employed to prevent the birth of an autistic child.

The objection to premise one is the claim that no one, not even parents, should have unchecked autonomy if their actions will result in harm to others. But perhaps the child, born autistic because his parents failed to use genetic technologies that would have prevented his birth, is not harmed by this action. Depending on the genetic technologies employed by the parents, the result may be that this child would not have been born at all. Would it not have been better for the child to be born autistic, than never to have been born at all? Such a claim follows from claims about the value of existence (Davis 2001; Buchanan et al. 2000). Surely it is better to exist at all, even with some disabilities, rather than to not exist. Granted, there may be some disabilities for which life with those disabilities is worse than never existing at all; however, autism is not one of those disabilities. One of the conclusions reached in chapter 2 is that we cannot dismiss the autistic person from moral consideration, as Benn might, even if the autistic person fails to have some traits that we associate with a good human life. The autistic person may not be living a full human life, given, for example, Nussbaum's claims about human capabilities, but it is better to exist with autism than never to have been born. We cannot say of the person born with a genetically transferable form of autism, "It would have been better for him had he not been born with autism," because in such a case that person would have been a different person altogether. The conclusion based on this line of reasoning is that parents are permitted to exercise their autonomy to allow a child to be born with autism, as the autistic child is not harmed by coming into existence when the alternative is never to have existed at all. In such a case, the objection to the first premise of the above argument is mistaken, and perhaps parents should have the last word when it comes to using—or not using—genetic technologies.

This conclusion may seem persuasive, but it is mistaken. It is wrong to claim that a life is better being actually lived than any other life that could possibly have been lived. It is true that it is better for a given person born with autism that his life is *better for him* than not existing at all. But prior to existing, it cannot be said of anyone that his life is better for him than not existing, because at that point, that individual does not exist (Parfit 1984). An example may be helpful in illustrating this point: John could say, "My life would have been so much better if I had not been born with psoriasis." John laments that his psoriasis is a congenital condition, and realizes that to lose this might entail losing some part of his genetic character, but he hates his psoriasis and wishes it were gone. His friends could respond by saying, "But if you had not been born that way, it would not have been you—it would have been someone else. In that case, you would never have existed, and we would have missed you terribly! This just goes to show that your psoriasis is really a good thing for you, after all." John's friends are claiming that an itchy skin condition is good, because they are comparing a life with psoriasis to no life at all. This is mistaken, though. They are right that without psoriasis, John may have been a different person; after all, psoriasis is a genetic condition, and once John's genetic makeup was sufficiently changed so as to prevent him from having that condition, other, more substantial changes may have ensued. But it is of course a mistake to conclude from the two alternatives—that one could either never exist at all, or exist with psoriasis—that psoriasis is good to have. For John, his life is good to have. A life without psoriasis would have been even better. Now that John exists, his existence is a good thing for him. But prior to his existence, his failure to exist did not hurt him, and his friends could hardly miss the John they never knew. The person who does not yet exist is not harmed or benefited by being brought into existence, for there is no one to either harm or benefit prior to the existence of that individual. The first premise of the argument from parental autonomy is false. Parental autonomy cannot be the last word in determining when genetic technologies may be used. A stronger argument must be found.

The Social Construction of Disability Argument

Another argument that says it is wrong to use genetic technologies to prevent the birth of children with disabilities is an argument that proceeds from the notion of a disability as socially constructed (Asch 1995). Rather than embrace a naturalistic model of disability, or one that is characterized by a notion of "harm," or "loss of freedom," or "loss of pleasure" (Gert et al. 1997), the argument that disability is socially constructed claims that were it not for social limitations imposed on those who have disabilities, the conditions that are called "disabling" might not be disabling at all. For example, in a society without staircases, persons unable to climb stairs would not be classified as disabled. The question of being unable to climb stairs would never be an issue in that society, any more than being unable to climb trees is considered a disability in our society. In a society that persists in creating staircases, individuals who cannot climb stairs are wrongly discriminated against as "disabled." Those of us unable to climb trees escape being labeled "disabled"; those who are unable to climb stairs carry that stigma. The labeling of individuals as "disabled" and discrimination against the disabled are of a piece: first, society notes certain features or characteristics that are undesirable; then society labels individuals as "disabled" based on those features or characteristics; and eventually parents are using genetic technologies to prevent the birth of a disabled child in a quest for the perfect baby. However there is nothing necessarily harmful in being disabled, if disability is merely socially constructed. Those of us who are unable to climb trees are not harmed by our incapacity, since our society exempts us from regularly performing this task. If we change society, we can change the harms that accrue to individuals in virtue of being labeled "disabled"; furthermore, these social barriers are well within our power to change (Asch 1995). Echoing this sentiment, Buchanan et al. say that we have an obligation to choose a communal arrangement "that is inclusive— that minimizes exclusion from participation on account of genetic impairments" (Buchanan et al. 2000, 20).

Given the social construction of disability, an argument against the use of genetic technologies to prevent the birth of persons with autism can be forwarded:

(1) Disabilities are socially constructed;

(2) If disabilities are socially constructed, then disabilities such as autism are not necessarily harmful to those persons who have them;

(3) If disabilities such as autism are not necessarily harmful to those who have them, then it not harmful to a person to be born with autism;

(4) If it is not harmful to a person to be born with autism, then parents should not use genetic technologies to prevent future children from being born with autism;

(5) Therefore, parents should not use genetic technologies to prevent future children from being born with autism.

Objections to this argument focus on premise one or premise three. Those who object to premise one, namely, "Disabilities are socially constructed," take issue with this claim. There are competing notions of the concepts of "disability," "disease," or "malady" which are not socially constructed. One claim is that these concepts are naturalistic; rather than being socially constructed, they are determined by the requirements of human functioning or survival (Caplan 1997). Naturalistic concepts of disease or disability claim that there is an objective fact, independent of society, which determines if a condition results in a disease, disability, or malady. Facts about human nature, human functioning, human survival, and human reproduction determine if a condition is in fact a disease or disability, not the dynamic nature of society (Steinbock 2000). Heart disease kills, and paralysis prevents you from moving—nothing about society will change these facts. An alternative conception of disease or disability is that these concepts are determined by conditions that result in harms such as losses of freedom or pleasure (Gert et al. 1997). Thus, it is not enough to say that the disability inherent in the inability to walk is merely socially constructed; there is a fact of the matter such that these conditions will result in a loss of opportunity for individuals. Even those who think that disability is socially constructed recognize that a significant physiological component exists in many cases (Asch 2000). Thus, the claim that disability is socially constructed is called into question, and the argument is determined to be unsound on the basis of a faulty claim in premise one.

A second objection to the argument is to grant that premise one is true, but to dispute premise three, namely, "If disabilities such as autism are not necessarily harmful to those who have them, then it not harmful to a person to be born with autism." It may be the case that disability is socially constructed to some degree, but the harms of being autistic will accrue to the person who is autistic in any case. The analogy between the person who cannot climb stairs and the person who does not have a functioning theory of mind fails. The absence of theory of mind dramatically affects the ability of the autistic individual to live a full life regardless of societal intervention. Some autistic individuals may develop "work around" strategies, learning by rote what comes naturally for persons with theory of mind. But while one can on the surface learn how to laugh when others laugh, or to embrace someone who starts to cry, without a fully functioning theory of mind there is still something missing. The complexities inherent in reciprocal human relationships, like the complexities inherent in the pragmatics of language mentioned by Lawson in chapter 3, cannot be learned by rote. A fundamental aspect of human relationships will always be missing for the person who does not have a functioning theory of mind. As observed in chapter 2, the lack of theory of mind limits the ability of the autistic person to enter into reciprocal relationships, which Nussbaum, Scanlon, Veatch, and Parfit argue is a fundamental part of a well-lived human life. Chapter 2 demonstrated that it is a philosophically risky strategy to pursue Benn's argument that the autistic individual is so far removed from other human beings that he is not part of the moral community. At the same time, given the limitations that result from being autistic, it is mistaken to say that the autistic individual is merely living a different kind of life, and if it were not for society's limitations, the autistic person would otherwise be fully integrated into society. Autistic individuals are not merely living a different kind of human life: the harms that accrue from being autistic are not merely the result of barriers constructed by society. There is something intrinsically limiting in an autistic life. The argument from the social construction of disabilities may hold with respect to some conditions, but it does not hold with respect to autism. For these reasons, the third premise is mistaken, and the argument from the social construction of disability is unsound.

The claim that the harms of autism were primarily socially constructed was at one time bolstered by the now discredited facilitated communication movement (American Academy of Pediatrics 1998). Erevelles (2002) examines the similarities between the social construction of other mental disorders and autism, as demonstrated by facilitated communication. To dispute the social construction of disability based on guilt-by-association is fallacious, however. The view can be dismissed on its own merits, and not merely based on its association with an unhappy chapter in the history of autism.

One argument closely related to the social construction of disability is the claim that preventing the birth of persons with disabilities will result in further discrimination against persons who are born with disabilities. There are two versions of this argument. The first is the "cumulative action" argument: as more parents find the means to prevent the birth of children with autism, there will be greater stigma in having autism for those few individuals who do have autism. Perhaps as there are fewer persons born with autism, there will be less funding for programs that are designed to help persons with autism. The "cumulative action" argument fails to take into consideration two points, however: not all cases of autism have a genetic component, so there will still be children born with autism even if genetic technologies to prevent the birth of some autistic persons becomes available. Second, individuals who are born with autism are born into individual families; while the birth of more persons with autism may prevent society from discriminating against persons with autism, it seems a tremendous burden to the individuals and their families to bear autism for the sake of changing the mind of others.

The second argument that preventing the birth of persons with a disability will result in greater discrimination against persons with disabilities is the "expressivist argument," which states that parents who decide not to have a child with a particular disability are sending the message that the disability in question is so terrible that a person is better off never having lived than living with that trait. In other words, the choice expresses bias and prejudice, thereby reinforcing discrimination against the disabled (Buchanan 1996; Parens and Asch 2000). Buchanan points out, however, that parents who knowingly prevent the birth of a child with disabilities may neither believe that the disability in question renders life not worth living, nor believe that only "perfect children" should be born (Buchanan 1996; Nelson 2000). Parents may simply believe that they are not prepared to care for a child with a particular disability, or that while there are some traits toward which the parents would be indifferent, the particular trait in question is not one that merits this indifference. But the belief that this disability is one that renders a life not worth living, or that the parents want a perfect child or none at all, may not be behind the parents' choice, and as such, the expressivist argument is also unsound.

The Deaf Community Argument and a Failed Analogy

Another argument against the use of genetic technologies to prevent the birth of persons with autism is the "Deaf community" argument (Davis 2001). Members of the Deaf community (uppercase "D," to designate the cultural understanding of deafness) have cited this argument against those who would use genetic technologies to prevent the birth of deaf (lowercase "d," to designate the physical condition of not being able to hear) children, or who would recommend the use of cochlear implants for children so that they could transition out of the Deaf community. The argument proceeds from the premise that there is a thriving Deaf community, and as such, to call anyone who is deaf and has the opportunity to join this community "disabled" is a misnomer. The Deaf community is comprised of deaf persons, has its own culture, its own languages, its own theater, norms, and values. The Deaf community argument is similar to the social construction of disability argument, in virtue of the fact that many Deaf people will say that given the choice, they would not elect to have hearing (Davis 2001). They do not identify deafness as a disability, and think that hearing persons' view about deafness as being a disability is merely a statement about the social construction of disability. The Deaf community argument then goes a step further than the social construction of disability argument: by asserting that there is a Deaf community of which deaf people can be a part, the Deaf community argument asserts not merely that the disability is socially constructed, but that there is a thriving social role for deaf individuals to occupy. The Deaf community is a vivid example of a close-knit community; there is also thriving Disability community, of which similar claims can be made (Asch 2000). It is possible to conclude that genetic technologies should not be employed to prevent the birth of persons with autism according to the following argument:

(1) Communities of persons with disabilities exist;
(2) If communities of persons with disabilities exist, then disabilities such as autism are not necessarily harmful to those persons who have them;

(3) If disabilities such as autism are not necessarily harmful to those who have them, then it not harmful to a person to be born with autism;

(4) If it is not harmful to a person to be born with autism, then parents should not use genetic technologies to prevent future children from being born with autism;

(5) Therefore, parents should not use genetic technologies to prevent future children from being born with autism.

The first premise could invoke the Deaf community, or any community of disabled persons, a community so rich that it is erroneous to call the members of the community "disabled." The Deaf community argument merely substitutes the word 'deaf' for the word 'autistic' in the above argument. But the Deaf community argument does not have a corollary for autistic persons—there is no Autistic community argument. What, after all, would it mean to talk about the Autistic community? One of the challenges facing individuals who lack a theory of mind is the failure to enter into reciprocal relationships. A community is not merely a collection of individuals who happen to have interests in common; rather, they have *common interests:* they share their interests, engage with each other, care for, or at the very least would care for each other were they aware of their commonality. The Autistic community is not merely those individuals who advocate on behalf of persons with autism. Unquestionably, in that sense, there is an Autistic community. Rather, the Autistic community should be understood as those individuals with autism, who have formed a community with other individuals with autism, just as the Deaf community is not merely those individuals who campaign on behalf of rights for the deaf, but who share community with the deaf. But the autistic individual, in virtue of a failure of theory of mind, does not have an analogous community.

A comparison between these types of communities and linguistic communities may be drawn. In chapter 1, Glüer and Pagin introduce the notion that autistic individuals can have "a kind of parasitic membership" in the linguistic community (Glüer and Pagin 2003). But this "parasitic membership" is not a sufficiently robust membership in a community needed for the above argument to be sound. The point of the argument is that having a community of persons with a given disability mitigates any shortcomings that might accrue from the disability itself. The "parasitic membership" that Glüer and Pagin cite—an individual riding other community members' coattails into the community—is not enough to qualify that individual for all of the goods that would counterbalance any drawbacks, socially constructed or otherwise, of the disability. The comparison only takes us so far: Glüer and Pagin are merely talking about a linguistic community, and not a full-fledged community filled with persons who share not only a language, but values, activities, and a culture. Even if autistic individuals could ride the coattails of other speakers into a shared linguistic community, this would not be enough to eventually forge an Autistic community.

An additional observation about autism and community can be gleaned from chapter 1's discussion of David Lewis's linguistic convention theory of meaning. For Lewis, *conventions*—including but not limited to linguistic conventions—are those practices that are *common knowledge* in a population. The examination of what constitutes *common knowledge* was shown to be problematic for autistic speakers who lacked a theory of mind. The conclusion in chapter 1 was that competent autistic speakers served as a counterexample to Lewis's theory of linguistic convention. Lewis might respond that individuals who are not able to tap into the common knowledge shared by a population are not actually members of that population. They may live among the members of the population, but not truly be members of that population in the ways that count. Of course, Lewis's position is one that defends only one concept of what it is to be a member of a given population, bound by conventions and common knowledge. The linguistic communities cited by Glüer and Pagin are also not sufficient to dismiss the possibility of an Autistic community.

Earlier claims about common interests and the way in which theory of mind deficits affect individuals' abilities to share common interests remain intact. Josef Parnas makes a similar point about schizophrenia. Parnas holds that schizophrenic hallucinations are distinct from other types of false beliefs, because they are typically not shared across individuals (Parnas 2004). Citing Karl Jaspers (1963), Parnas explains that persons with schizophrenic hallucinations "are detached due to their idiosyncratic affective valence, the themes are not really about the common world, and the patient does not expect similar tribulations to affect his fellow humans. It is for these reasons that the schizophrenic patients never construct a true 'societas schizophren-ica'" (Parnas 2004, 158). But while there are similarities, the cases are not identical. The person experiencing hallucinations may not hold that others have the same beliefs, but he does recognize the full personhood—including rich intentional ascriptions not hamstrung by a unified consciousness view—of the others who have beliefs which are at variance with his own. The person with autism's difficulty is more profound, making the possibility of engaging in and identifying with a community more daunting. Thus, premise two of the above argument is mistaken. While it is true that communities of persons exist, both disabled and otherwise, it is not the case that a community of autistic persons is one of them. There is not, nor could there be, a community of autistic persons, since a failure of theory of mind would preclude being a part of a community in a fundamental sense.

One objection to this line of reasoning states that it does not always follow from the epistemic point that *something is not known to exist,* or that *something is not recognized to exist* that *it in fact does not exist.* There are buried rocks no one has uncovered, long-lost love letters hidden in attics, and far-off celestial bodies yet to be discovered. All of these exist, even if they are not known to or recognized to exist. There are some cases, however, in which knowing a thing exists is a necessary condition for that thing to exist. This is true of community. Someone who lacks theory of mind does not merely fail to recognize that he has a community from which he is estranged. Rather, without a theory of mind one of the basic building blocks of a community is something of which an agent is wholly unaware: the agent does not know that there are others out there such that a community is a possibility. The person who lacks a theory of mind does not claim, "I might have a community out there, I just do not know where they are, or I do not know where to find them." For the person who lacks a theory of mind there is no *they,* there is no *them.* There are not persons in the rich sense that would be needed in order to share in a genuine community. The autistic person is unlike the racist who might say, "I know who my community is, but I am not a part of *your* community, nor are you a part of *mine.*" The racist is someone who does recognize that he belongs to a community, and knows what it is to be a member of a community, but he has misguided views as to what the relevant criteria are to determine what constitutes true community. The racist fails to see that he actually is a part of a community that he abhors, but he is unlike the person with autism: the person with autism does not say, "I reject this community *qua* community and instead embrace a different community."

Perhaps the autistic person would recognize his community, if only he did not have a compromised theory of mind. But the whole point of theory of mind deficits is that the lack of theory of mind is a fundamental deficit that is characteristic of autism: if he did not have a compromised theory of mind, he would not be autistic. Thus, the claim "If he did not have a compromised theory of mind, he would recognize X as his community, and thus X is his community" does not make sense.

A final point arises when considering the unique theory of mind deficits that the autistic person encounters in the context of using genetic technologies to prevent the birth of children with autism. It has been argued that parents should look past the disabilities that their children may face, and instead focus on the relationships that they can have with their children: "Good parents will care about raising whatever child they receive and about the relationship that will develop, not about the traits that the child bears" (Parens and Asch 2000, 18). But as discussed in chapter 2, serious questions about this relationship emerge. Autism is unique from any physical or mental disability, in that it affects the nature of relationships. To grant this point, and to claim that parents should care about the relationship that emerges, no matter how compromised it is, glosses over many of the points made in chapter 2.

All of the above arguments—the parental autonomy argument, the social construction of disability argument, and the Deaf community argument—come up short in their attempts to demonstrate that it is not morally acceptable to use genetic technologies to prevent the birth of persons with autism. An argument that attempts to show that it is morally acceptable to use genetic technologies to prevent the birth of persons with autism is one based on a familiar concept in moral and legal philosophy: the right to an open future.

Autism and the Right to an Open Future

Arguments for the permissibility to use genetic technologies from the right to an open future are well known (Davis 2001). The right to an open future was first articulated by Joel Feinberg as a means of understanding autonomy rights that are held in trust for persons who do not yet have autonomy, but one day will be autonomous agents (Feinberg 1980). Individuals who will eventually have autonomy, such as children, should have that future autonomy preserved, even if it does not yet exist. It is wrong to perform an action that would violate a person's right to an open future, even if that person does not yet have autonomy, and even if that person's present autonomy is not compromised by that action. For example, it is wrong for parents to sterilize an eight-year-old girl. The eight-year-old is not pregnant today, nor is it expected that she would be pregnant any time soon. It can be argued that the child is not harmed today by being sterilized. But it is reasonable to assume that eventually she may wish to become pregnant based on an autonomous choice, and that the parents' actions today would restrict her from being able to make this autonomous choice later on. It is harmful to perform an action that would eventually harm her future autonomy, such as sterilizing her at a young age. This is an example of parents violating a child's right to an open future: their actions would close doors of possibility for the child, restricting her ability to act autonomously later in life.

It is wrong for parents to violate a child's right to an open future. Of course it is inevitable that some actions taken by parents to promote the right to an open future will also result in curtailing the child's open future in some respects: sending a child to one school invariably prevents him from attending another school, thereby closing off some doors of possibility in an attempt to open others. One school may have an excellent science program, a different school may have a world-class foreign language program. Parents must choose between them, and creating one set of opportunities necessarily closes the door on the others. Parents cannot be faulted for closing some doors in an attempt to open others. Rather, it is wrong to act in such a way that knowingly prevents a maximal number of doors of possibility to be open, or to close off those doors of possibility that affect a child's future right to make autonomous choices. The maximal number of doors of possibility should not be understood merely in terms of quantity of options, but also in terms of quality, and the ability to allow the child to pursue his interests autonomously.

Sometimes it is difficult to know if the doors of possibility are opening or closing: how does a parent know when the choice to send a child to an elite boarding school restricts or upholds the right to an open future? On one hand, the child may be getting a tremendous education, far better than the education available locally. On the other hand, the child may benefit from being at home with the family, and the local educational opportunities may be strong in their own right. Which group of friends would be better for the child—and how could one possibly know? In some cases the right to an open future may raise more questions than it answers. In other cases, the call is an easy one. It is a violation of the eight-year-old's right to an open future to be sterilized; it is a violation of the right to an open future for a child to be born autistic. Being autistic limits your life chances in numerous ways. As discussed in chapter 2, philosophers such as Nussbaum, Scanlon, Veatch, and Parfit believe that having relationships with other persons is a significant part of what makes a human life go well. Benn goes so far as to say that the absence of reactive attitudes disqualifies a person from moral agency. Benn holds the most radical position, but even those who take a more moderate view recognize that being autistic compromises a person's ability to live the fullest human life.

From the concept of a right to an open future, an argument in favor of using genetic technologies to prevent the birth of children with autism would follow:

(1) Parents are not morally permitted to knowingly restrict their child's right to an open future;

(2) Having autism restricts a child's right to an open future;

(3) Therefore, parents are not morally permitted to knowingly have a child with autism;

(4) Genetic technologies may one day be available that will allow parents to avoid having children with autism;

(5) Therefore, parents should use genetic technologies, if they one day become available, to avoid having children with autism.

The argument relies heavily on the right to an open future: if this right is called into question, then the first premise is false and the argument is unsound. Thus, a further examination of the right to an open future is warranted.

One concern is that the right to an open future is an imprecise standard—as stated above, it is difficult for parents to know if a particular course of action will uphold or restrict a child's right to an open future. There are two responses to this objection. The first is to say that while it is certainly difficult to know when the right to an open future is compromised, that does not change the fact that it is a parent's obligation to uphold it. Parents cannot be held blameworthy for the failure to perform an action that upheld their children's right to an open future, especially when they did their best to investigate all of their options, and acted in a way that by all appearances was consistent with their child's interests. But even if the parents are not blameworthy for a failure to uphold their child's right to an open future, this does not change the fact that the parents have this obligation, and that in retrospect it would have been better had they acted in such a way that better upheld their child's right. After doing all the research that they could, parents might send their child to the boarding school, only to realize later that this was the wrong choice. Even though the parents could not have known otherwise, the course of action may still be wrong, as parents who admit "It would have been better had we done so-and-so" acknowledge. The right to an open future is not seriously challenged by the fact that it is difficult to know which course of action best upholds the standard.

The second response to the claim that the right to an open future is an imprecise standard is to concede that there are often grey areas in which it is difficult to know when the right to an open future is being compromised, or in which the alternatives available appear to equally maintain the right to an open future. Asch argues this very point:

> The child who will have a disability may have fewer options for the so-called open future that philosophers and parents dream of for a child. Yet I suspect that disability precludes far fewer life possibilities than members of the bioethics community claim. (Asch 1999, 528)

Asch cites several examples: a wheelchair may preclude mountain climbing, but not all athletic activities; Down syndrome does not preclude thinking, analysis, or creativity; and so on. Asch is right that we ought not be too hasty in dismissing a life that precludes an open future. However, the case of autism is not one of these grey cases. Given that autism limits the ability of a person to have reciprocal relationships with others, one of the essential elements of a well-lived human life, it does not make sense to say that, *ceteris paribus,* there are as many doors of possibility open, or that the doors available are just as conducive to promoting a child's future, whether a child is autistic or not.

A second concern with the right to an open future is that it creates a standard that is too far-reaching in terms of which genetic conditions parents must work to prevent. There would seem to be innumerable genetic conditions that would limit a child's right to an open future. Are parents required to act to prevent future children from having every one of these conditions? Rather than embracing the right to an open future as a standard for parents to determine when it is permissible or obligatory to employ genetic technologies, other philosophers have drawn the line elsewhere. Laura Purdy says that we have an obligation to provide for future persons a "minimally satisfying life" (Purdy 2006, 529). It is difficult to pin down what a "minimally satisfying life" might consist in, although it would appear to only create an obligation on the part of parents to avoid the most devastating genetic conditions. Anything less than an extreme case would seem to qualify as a "minimally satisfying life," including a life with autism. If what Purdy means by a "minimally satisfying life" is that we should avoid bringing persons into existence whose lives are worse than not existing at all, a life with autism meets Purdy's standard. Purdy mentions a life with Huntington's disease as an example of a life that fails to be "minimally satisfying"; it would seem that she draws the line somewhat higher than at a life that is no better than no life at all. Ronald M. Green says that parents have a *prima facie* obligation to "not bring a child into being deliberately or negligently with a health status likely to result in significantly greater disability or suffering, or significantly reduced life options relative to the other children with whom he/she will grow up" (Green 1997, 10). This is not so much a standard as a moving target, as different birth cohorts will result in different claims about what is permissible; however, it is certainly the case that an autistic child is not as well off as the child's birth cohort. The point here is that the right to an open future is not the only standard available to those who would make the argument that parents have the obligation to employ genetic technologies to prevent their children from having autism: Purdy's claim would be that a life with autism is not "minimally satisfying," and Green's claim is that a life with autism is not as good as one shared by the child's birth cohort. Although one standard is highly objective and the other is relativistic, Purdy and Green are in agreement when it comes to autism. However, Purdy's standard, while objective, is difficult to define, and the flexibility of Green's standard may be ultimately unsatisfying.

It is possible to view the right to an open future as an attempt to split the difference between Purdy's and Green's two standards: finding a middle ground between an objective, but vague standard, and a relativistic, but clearly defined standard. It is not the case that the right to an open future standard is merely an attempt to split the difference—it has merits in its own right. However, the right to an open future standard does incorporate some of the virtues of both Purdy's and Green's standards, while eschewing some of the more problematic aspects. Like Purdy's standard, the right to an open future attempts to generate an objective standard about what is required of parents when providing for their children. Like Green's cohort standard, the right to an open future presents more than a minimalist requirement for what parents owe their future children.

A final objection to the right to an open future standard is that it is a peculiarly liberal standard, relying too much on the principle of autonomy (Davis 2001). William Ruddick finds the right to an open future an "ultraliberal standard" which he modifies into a "life-options provision principle":

> Roughly, my idea is that parents must help foster a range of life prospects or life options for a child, any one of which would be acceptable to both parents and child if realized. Conversely, they need not foster any life option that they themselves would find unacceptable if taken up by their child. Nor may they force a life prospect on a child that the child could be predicted in its maturity to reject. (Ruddick 2000, 101)

Rather than focus solely on the child's future autonomous choices, this standard looks to a mutually acceptable life plan as autonomously chosen by both the parents and the child, once he or she becomes autonomous. This tempering of the right to an open future does not entirely address the objection that the principle is too focused on autonomy, however. After all, Ruddick's suggestion simply adds the parents' autonomous choices into the mix, along with the child's autonomous choices. As long as the child enters a mutually agreed-upon open door, Ruddick's position is indistinguishable from the right to an open future. And if no mutually agreed-upon door exists? Whose choices should then carry the day? In such a case, it should be the child's future autonomous choices that should determine what should be done, as he or she will be the one who is most affected by those life choices. At this point, the right to an open future is again the principle by which parents should make their choices.

A variation on the objection that the right to an open future is too liberal is that it does not make sufficient use of other bioethical principles, such as beneficence, nonmaleficence, or justice, and instead places too much emphasis on autonomy. The right to an open future tempers unchecked autonomy on the part of parents against the future autonomy of the child. This reining-in of parental autonomy by the autonomy of future persons may actually be an advantage of the right to an open future: rather than attempting to claim that another principle should trump autonomy in this case, the right to an open future holds a single principle of value. However, there may be other disadvantages to the reliance on the principle of autonomy. With respect to cases of autism, this liberal standard seems particularly confounding. As discussed in chapter 3, one of the difficulties the autistic person faces is that many moral theories are non-starters for persons lacking a functioning theory of mind. Liberal theories, which place tremendous value on autonomy rights of individuals, are problematic to apply to the person with autism. The liberal's own rights are of tremendous value, but the liberal is also bound to respect the rights of others. Without a fully functioning theory of mind, the autistic person moves in a world of action without volition—persons do things, but a full understanding of these individuals as autonomous beings with their own intentional states is lacking. There are many competing analyses of the concept of "autonomy" (Beauchamp and Childress 2001; Dworkin 1988; O'Neill 2002), but all of them share ascriptions of intentionality to those individuals who possess autonomy.

Another problem with the right to an open future is that this standard seems to be very much in keeping with an ethic of *prima facie* duties, such as Beauchamp and Childress's principles of biomedical ethics. In chapter 3 it was shown that an ethic of *prima facie* duties is not one that would be readily embraced by persons with autism. The trade-offs between autonomy, future autonomy, beneficence, and nonmaleficence that characterize the right to an open future may not be persuasive to persons with autism, as argued by Lawson. Neither the intuitively motivated principles themselves, nor the intuitively motivated balancing of the principles are compelling to the person who lacks a theory of mind.

The upshot is that non-autistic persons may embrace the liberal right to an open future, recognizing the inherent autonomy of others, but the liberal right to an open future can be baffling to a person lacking theory of mind. The right to an open future provides us with a standard for using genetic technologies that would require parents to prevent the birth of autistic persons, but it is a standard that autistic persons might not understand, let alone agree with.[6] As seen in chapter 3, many moral theories leave autistic and non-autistic people talking past each other. Applied questions in ethics leave us in no better shape.

It is possible to object to premise two of the argument, namely, "Having autism restricts a child's right to an open future," based on the following line of reasoning: it can be agreed that it is better that fewer children are born with autism, and that having autism restricts an individual's opportunities, but it is a mistake to claim that *having a property* restricts a person's *rights*. There are two versions of this objection. The first is that possessing properties themselves do not uphold, nor do they undermine, a person's rights. Actions performed by agents can uphold or undermine a person's rights, but properties that agents possess cannot. This objection fails to recognize that what parents are doing in allowing a child to be born with autism is *performing an action* that will result in a person having a particular property. It is imprecise to say "autism restricts a child's right to an open future" when strictly speaking "a parent's action that results in a child being born with autism restricts that child's right to an open future." Brevity may be the soul of many things, but clear philosophical arguments are often spirited away without this asset.

The second version of this objection is to challenge the notion of a "right," claiming that there are no actions that are *prima facie* right or wrong such that it is a violation of an individual's rights to perform those actions. There is a long utilitarian tradition of not recognizing rights (Ross 2002; Sen 1991), or working diligently to try to accommodate rights into utilitarian theories which appear, on their face, to not recognize rights (Brandt 1992; Frey 1984). Those responding to this objection are left to make sense of the right to an open future in the absence of "rights." The best recourse for the utilitarian is to argue that the right to an open future is a method by which parents forestall performing some actions that will affect utilities for their children, with the expectation that utilities will be maximized if the child ultimately performs those actions himself. There are some cases in which a parent has no choice but to act now to try to maximize utilities in the long run, but there are other cases—enrolling a child in a school that will give him a broad liberal education rather than a professional school that will prepare him for a single career—designed to keep as many doors open to utility maximization as possible. Those cases in which the parents act to keep as many options open for a child, so that the child may eventually perform actions that will maximize utility, are cases in which parents are acting in keeping with the "right" to an open future, even if recognizing that no such "right" exists.

But even if this strategy is pursued, as seen in chapter 3, utilitarianism may not be persuasive to the person with autism, either. This strategy may be persuasive to the person without autism, but these positions will not be compelling to the person who lacks a theory of mind, and in virtue of that, may not find utility maximization a moral imperative.

A final objection may point to the argument's strong conclusion: according to this argument it is not merely the case that parents are permitted to use genetic technologies to prevent the birth of a child with autism; rather, they *should* do this, they are *obligated* to do this. A failure to use genetic technologies, should they become available, is a failure to uphold a fundamental right of one's future children. Objecting to the conclusion is not an option when attempting to find an argument unsound. One of the premises must be mistaken if the argument is unsound—simply stating that the conclusion is too strong is not an objection. As the argument stands, it is the case that parents are obligated to do what they can to prevent the birth of an autistic child. One means by which parents who are at risk of having a child with autism may accomplish this is to consider sex selection. A discussion of this option is presented below.

Using Sex Selection to Prevent
the Birth of Autistic Persons

Given the sizable male-to-female ratio among persons with autism, one question that might be asked is whether it is permissible to use sex selection to prevent the birth of a child with autism. No one knows at present which genes result in autism, but we do know that autism is far more likely to affect males than females. It is estimated that there is a four-to-one ratio of boys to girls with autism, and as high as a fifteen-to-one ratio of boys to girls with Asperger's syndrome (Frith 2003). It is unknown whether being male makes someone more vulnerable to autism, or if being female constitutes a protective advantage, but the overwhelming ratio of males to females with autism is not in dispute. One hypothesis discussed briefly in chapter 1 is that autism is an extreme form of the male brain, more attuned to systematizing than to empathizing, which explains why more males are autistic than females (Baron-Cohen 2003).

As discussed earlier in this chapter, current evidence for a genetic component to autism is primarily based on family histories. Some families may recognize themselves to be at risk for having an autistic child, given autism in their extended family, or given that the family already has one autistic child (Baron-Cohen 2000a). At present, if a family has a child with autism the likelihood that they will have a second child with autism "is 2 to 6 percent—about 100 times the general risk" (Goode 2004b). Parents in these circumstances may have good reason to believe that their likelihood of having a child with autism is decreased if they have a female child. Having a female child is no guarantee that the child will not have autism, it merely reduces that possibility. There is presently no identified gene for autism that is necessarily linked to the X chromosome. Identification of, for example, a fetus with Fragile X syndrome, could be viewed very differently than a fetus which is more likely to have autism simply by virtue of being male. Thomas H. Murray, while disagreeing with sex selection, nonetheless quotes the Council of International Organizations for Medical Science's 1990 Working Group on Genetic Screening and Testing, which eschewed sex selection "other than to avoid X-linked diseases" (Murray 1996, 126). While Fragile X syndrome raises the likelihood that a child will have autism, Fragile X is a disorder in its own right. But what if there is no condition, such as Fragile X, that has been identified? Rather, all that is known is that the rate of autism among males is greater than among females. Is it morally permissible, given this fact, to select the sex of a future child in an attempt to prevent the birth of a child with autism?

While parental autonomy would seem to argue in favor of the permissibility of sex selection, some philosophers have argued against using sex selection. The arguments against unchecked parental autonomy, presented earlier in this chapter, are employed in this case: unchecked autonomy is not permissible when it comes to making choices for a child, including choosing the sex of a future child. Another argument against sex selection is a population-based argument: the population as a whole would suffer if sex selection were permitted to occur. The overwhelming cases of sex selection globally involve parents choosing to have male children over female. For this reason, if widespread sex selection were allowed to occur, a large-scale imbalance of one sex over the other would result. This imbalance would result in unrest and unhappiness; thus, sex selection should not be permitted (Davis 2001). Yet another argument is an argument based upon bias: given the larger number of cases of sex selection in favor of males and against females, allowing sex selection will perpetuate bias against females. Kittay observes, "In racism and pernicious nationalism, the exclusive appropriation of desirable properties is usually tied to restrictions on reproduction" (Kittay 2005, 120)—just as restrictions on reproduction have followed from claims about the superiority of one race or nationality, similar claims about the superiority of one gender over the other are perpetuated with sex selection. This is a version of the expressivist argument mentioned earlier in this chapter, but applied in this case to questions of sex rather than disability (Parens and Asch 2000). Both the population-based argument and the expressivist argument are compelling, but are compelling only in cases in which many, many parents use sex selection (Zilberberg 2004). In the case of parents who are at risk of having an autistic child, such concerns are not relevant—it is not the case that large numbers of families are known to be at risk for autism at the time such choices are made. It should also be noted that although the population-based argument and the expressivist argument apply to cases in which parents are selecting *for* male children, and the families who are at risk for autism are selecting *against* male children, this fact is irrelevant. The population-based argument and the expressivist argument would be just as sound if parents overwhelmingly chose females: the same consequences of unrest, unhappiness, or bias would ensue. However, these arguments are not relevant to the comparatively isolated cases of sex selection to prevent the birth of an autistic child.

A compelling argument against sex selection is an argument from the right to an open future: children who are born to parents who selected their sex will be under undue expectations based upon their gender. The argument proceeds from the assumption that parents who care enough to select the sex of their child are more likely to have strong expectations about gender roles—why else would they care so much about having a child of the "right" gender? Claims such as "having a boy will balance out the family" or "I've always wanted a girl" carry implicit expectations about what being a boy or girl means, and what a person occupying these roles will bring to a family (Barnbaum 2001). Having to live out these roles, especially after having being selected with these roles in mind, may compromise a child's right to an open future, once again closing those doors of opportunity. Of course these roles may be imposed on a child even if that child's sex is not chosen, but allowing the parents to choose the child's sex will only exacerbate an already difficult situation in that case. As such, sex selection should not be permitted.[7]

The right to an open future cuts both ways in this case: just as it may restrict parents from choosing the sex of their child in most cases, it allows for sex selection in the case of families that are at risk for autism. A child with autism has a future that is less open than that of a child who did not have autism, *ceteris paribus*. So the right to an open future seems to imply that sex selection is both permissible and impermissible. How are these two positions reconciled? Both positions can be reconciled once it is recognized that there are some circumstances (growing up with strong gender expectations) that are not *as limiting* as others (growing up with autism). While the limitations placed on a person by strong gender expectations should not be dismissed, those restrictions are not nearly as wide-ranging as those that result from autism. Autism severely compromises one's right to an open future, more so than strong gender expectations. Furthermore, at-risk families that choose female children over male children are not choosing females because of a specific gender role; they are choosing a female child to prevent the likelihood that their future child has autism (Zilberberg 2004; Steinbock 2002). In light of this, at-risk families may be limiting their child's right to an open future minimally, if at all, by choosing a female child over a male child. However, while such a choice may limit that child's right to an open future slightly, a far more significant limitation will ensue if the parents have a child with autism. Thus parents who know they are at risk for having a child who is autistic should take advantage of sex selection when they can as a small step to prevent the birth of a child with autism. It is not merely morally permissible to use sex selection in such a case; it may be morally obligatory in an attempt to promote what is best for future children.

Objections to this claim emerge from the fact that choosing a female child does not guarantee that the child will not have autism, and that some methods of sex selection may be less than 100 percent successful. Thus, the following scenario might emerge: parents of a son with autism know that they are at risk for having a second child with autism. They opt for sex selection, hoping for a female child who may be less likely to be autistic, although no guarantees are available. The parents' plan may be thwarted in two ways. In one case, the woman becomes pregnant, but owing to the error rate of the sex selection technology, she becomes pregnant with a male child. In the second case the woman becomes pregnant with the desired female child, and months after she is born it is discovered that the daughter has autism. Given the possibility of failure, are parents harming their future children, or themselves, by using these technologies? Might it do more harm than good to choose a child with particular traits only to have those expectations frustrated? Parents who did what they could to prevent the birth of a child with autism, but who nonetheless had a child with autism, may be all the more heartbroken. Perhaps it would have been better to not try to avoid autism at all, than to try, only to have those expectations undermined.

This objection is not persuasive, as it would prove too much. If it is wrong to take actions to promote the good for future children, because in some cases the results are less than hoped-for, then it similarly would be wrong to take folic acid to prevent neural-tube defects, or to abstain from alcohol while pregnant in order to prevent brain damage to future children. Some children of women who do take folic acid have neural tube defects, and some children of women who abstain from alcohol while pregnant have brain damage. The failure in some cases does not undermine the good of the action when it achieves the desired result. Thus, parents should continue to do the best they can for their future children, even in cases where there is no guarantee that their actions will have the intended result. In the small percentage of cases in which parents already know they are at risk for having a child with autism, sex selection is presently their best option, both medically and morally.

A final consideration emerges: there is some evidence that girls with autism do more poorly than boys with autism (Bazelon 2007; Howlin et al. 2004). If this true, then the sex selection question is confounded by a trade-off for high-risk families between a greater likelihood that a child will be born with autism, albeit a less severe case, and a small likelihood that a child will be born with autism, but one with considerably fewer opportunities. What should be done under those circumstances? It is hard to pose the question without inevitable comparisons to expected utility, raising the same objections posed by Nussbaum and Kittay at the beginning of chapter 2. Nussbaum, Kittay, and others would object to human lives being measured via expected utility, where more people with less profound disabilities are weighed against fewer people with more profound disabilities. Understandably, this type of cost-benefit analysis is repugnant to some. For others, the cost-benefit is not merely repugnant, but absurd: each future child is the only one living his or her own life. What does it even mean for each individual person to compare his or her life to the life of a mere possible human being who never existed?

Replying to this objection involves taking a close look at autism and the nature of autistic deficits. Autism cuts people off from people, undermining reciprocal relationships. As a society, we expect women to both value and to engage in reciprocal relationships to a greater degree than men. A man who has lived alone all his life, eats the same meals on the same days of the week, and obsessively maps medieval fantasy worlds is a quirky loner. The woman who has lived alone all of her life, has the same eating habits, and obsessively blogs fan fiction about the same medieval fantasy world is viewed far more negatively. This is where Asch's points about the social construction of disability have merit. Given the distinct expectations of women and men in our society, a woman *qua* woman may be more harmed by theory of mind deficits than a man would be. Asch is right, however: this inequity is within society's power to change. Theory of mind deficits are devastating to everyone who suffers them, as illustrated in chapter 2's observations about the importance of relationships in a good human life. But to say that women are even more damaged by theory of mind deficits than men may be predicated on societal expectations of women's friendships, or the significance of relationships in a woman's world. Women with autism may further internalize this, asking why they cannot be more like Jane Austin's heroines. The barriers to becoming like Daniel Defoe's heroes are not inherent in the nature of autism. *These* expectations *are* within our power to change.

Voices of Autism

Temple Grandin *is a full professor of animal sciences at Colorado State University. She established a national reputation designing cattle chutes and slaughterhouses, designs that both reduce animal stress and promote the humane slaughter of animals. In addition to her work in animal sciences, Dr. Grandin is known for her publications and lectures on her experiences with autism. In the second of her autobiographical books,* Thinking in Pictures and Other Reports from My Life with Autism, *she discusses animal science, autism, as well as the ways in which autism has contributed to a richer understanding of her profession.*

Her essays range over a variety of topics, including the way in which autism results in her pictorial way of thinking, the role of emotions in her life, and human relationships. Grandin credits her pictorial way of thinking for her abilities to design humane cattle-processing plants, as well as her ability to draw complex diagrams of her designs with little formal drafting education. Grandin only recently came to appreciate that her way of thinking is dramatically different from other people. Not everyone who has autism possesses this pictorial way of thinking, but Grandin believes that in her case the two are linked. "I would never want to become so normal that I would lose those skills," she says (Grandin 1995, 180).

Another of Grandin's notable inventions is her "squeeze machine," created to replicate the sensation of being hugged without human contact. All her life Grandin avoided being touched by other people, yet sought the comforting feeling of being hugged. Sensory difficulties made hugs from other people too uncomfortable. Her first experience simulating hugs was to get inside a cattle chute at her aunt's ranch. Since that time Grandin has modified and redesigned squeeze machines of her own making which simulate the feeling of being hugged, as well as relieve fear and anxiety (Grandin 1995, 63).

Despite the assertion that "Fortunately, none of my siblings are autistic" (Grandin 1995, 176), Grandin does not want to be "cured" of the condition that makes her who she is. She reiterates sentiments from chapter 3, saying that she ". . . would not want to lose my ability to think visually. I have found my place along the great continuum" (Grandin 1995, 60–61).

5

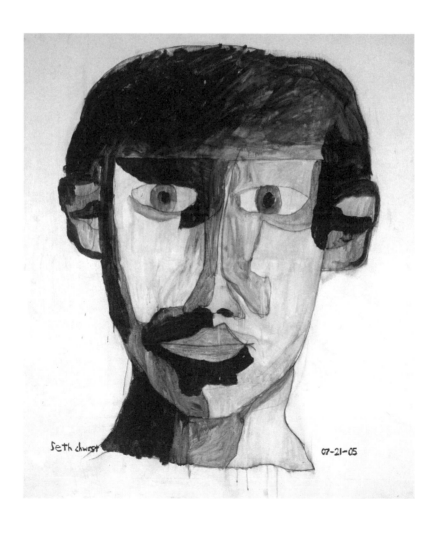

SETH CHWAST, *SELF-STUDY IN SLATE BLUE*

Research on Persons with Autism

Human subjects research raises significant questions. Is it ever permissible to use human beings as research subjects? If it is permissible, is it ever permissible to use human beings who are not competent decision makers as research subjects? The particulars of the answer to both questions—what makes human subjects research permissible at all, and what is the basis for appropriate proxy decisions—are the focus of this chapter.

Research on autism can take two forms. Given the genetic basis of some cases of autism, some research on the causes of autism will necessarily include research into extended families, searching for possible genetic precursors (Chen et al. 2003). Research on autism, especially on the families of children with autism, has a history that is particularly fraught. At one time parents, and in particular the mothers of children with autism, were believed to cause the condition in their children. These claims were based on mistaken assumptions about cause and effect, the toll that having a child with autism take on family members, as well as sampling errors (Kotsopoulos 2000). Blaming parents for their child's autism is a pernicious practice. Yet even today it persists, in the guise of misplaced admonitions that parents should not have vaccinated their child, should alter their child's diet, or are not engaging in therapeutic play of sufficient quality or quantity.[1] Researchers should be cognizant that many parents of children with autism are aware of this painful history; thus researchers should guard against the perception that research into the family history of autism can, or will, be used to impart blame. When researching genetic precursors of any disease, it is inevitable that some guilt may emerge on the part of family members. But given the mistakes and abuses that surround autism, researchers should be particularly sensitive on this count.

Family members may or may not have autism themselves, but they may carry genes that could contribute to autism. In some instances, the results of those genetic precursors may not be harmful to the person who carries them. For example, among fathers of people with autism who were particularly good at detail-oriented tasks, the fathers' attention to detail "resembled individuals with autism, but, importantly, for these fathers their detail-focused cognitive style was an asset not a deficit" (Happé 2000, 212). Family members who do not have autism and are competent decision makers are in a position to give informed consent to participate in research. For non-autonomous family members, such as young siblings of persons with autism, care must be taken that appropriate surrogate consent and other research protections are in place.

Several types of harms can accrue to otherwise healthy family members who participate in research into autism's genetic aspects. First, it is possible that a family member could be found to carry genes that put that individual at risk of having a child with autism, knowledge that may bring stress and anxiety. Potential parents, knowing that they carry genetic precursors to autism, may find that knowledge a substantial burden, forcing them to grapple with many of the issues considered in the previous chapter. Second, it is possible that this information could put individuals' insurability in jeopardy. While some genetic precursors to autism may not be directly harmful, and may even be beneficial to individuals who posses them, the fact that their future children are at greater risk for autism may disqualify the parents, or future children, from some insurance policies. As discussed in the beginning of chapter 4, the costs of raising a child with autism are substantial. Third, a problem of distributive justice emerges when families of persons with autism are asked to be research subjects. Family members may be asked, time and again, to participate in studies designed to learn about autism, a burden that escapes families without autistic members. In addition to the above problems, family members may be taken advantage of due to the desperation they might experience by virtue of taking care of a person with autism, or the unrealistic hope that research participation will result in direct benefits to their autistic family member (Chen et al. 2003). These considerations should be weighed off against the fact that family members may find research participation gratifying, in light of the paucity of options available to help their autistic family member.

The second form of research into autism uses individuals who have autism as subjects. This research can range broadly. One type includes *behavioral research* described in chapter 1, such as the Sally-Anne or Smarties false-belief tasks. A second type of research on persons with autism includes *minimally invasive research,* such as genetic research that might involve blood draws, which involves only minimal risk.² A third type is research that could include *both minimal risk aspects and more invasive aspects, but which is not aimed at curing* persons with autism, only relieving them of some of the more trying symptoms of the disorder. In particular, many persons with autism describe sensory difficulties. Bright lights or colors, high-pitched sounds, or scratchy clothing are repeatedly described by persons with autism as painful, sometimes to the point of being excruciating. The validity of these self-reports is the basis of the debate in chapter 1 between Frith and Happé on one hand, and McGeer on the other. McGeer argues that these reports of painful sensory experiences should be taken at face value, whereas Frith and Happé disagree, using such accounts as one basis for calling into question the ability of autistic persons to reflect accurately on their own internal states. If McGeer is correct, then we should take very seriously the cacophony of sensory overload experienced by persons with autism. Research into these problems aims not at a cure, but at an alleviation of symptoms. Treatments for these problems would be the equivalent of wearing sunglasses on a particularly bright day: blocking out some of the visual light actually enables the wearer to see more clearly. However, as argued later, even this seemingly straightforward point is confounded by the complexity of autism.

Finally, research on persons with autism could include *invasive biomedical research.* The focus of this chapter is on more controversial biomedical research, primarily research that is aimed at "curing" autism, as opposed to merely relieving some of its symptoms. Studies on potential "cures" for autism will necessarily involve using persons who have autism as research participants. A small minority of persons with high-functioning autism may be competent to offer informed consent to participate in some of these research projects. Questions still remain, however, about the ethical protections for persons with autism who are not competent to consent on their own behalf. Bioethicists have thoroughly investigated the use of less-than-autonomous research subjects in biomedical research. However, the unique nature of the deficits faced by persons with autism challenges some of the well-known claims about the use of non-competent autistic research subjects.

This chapter examines the ethics of using persons with autism in biomedical research. The first set of questions examines the use of persons with autism in research at all—how do the canonical arguments for and against the use of human research subjects fare when considering persons with autism? The second set of questions examines standards of proxy decision making that are employed when making decisions on behalf of less-than-autonomous research subjects. One standard—the substituted judgment standard—is not applicable to incompetent persons with autism. The second standard—the best interest standard—is applicable, but only up to a point. There is one significant case in which the best interest standard fails. This chapter concludes with a call for autistic integrity—a recognition that adults with autism should be treated with respect, which may preclude their participation in research studies that might aim to "cure" them of theory of mind disorders.

Kantian Arguments, Utilitarian Arguments, Principlism, and Autism

Before asking what justifies using persons with autism in medical research, a question can be asked as to whether it is *ever* permissible to use human beings in medical research. This question is especially crucial in cases in which the persons are unable to consent to participate in research on their own behalf. Three familiar arguments have been posited—two in favor of the use of human research subjects, and one against. The force of both arguments is tempered in light of the ethical implications of autism.

One argument cited in favor of using persons as research subjects is a utilitarian argument: utility is maximized when persons are used as research subjects, thus human subjects research is morally permissible (Barnbaum and Byron 2001). Unchecked act-utilitarianism is rarely invoked to justify the use of human research subjects, as this could result in research performed without informed consent or other valuable protections. However, with those protections in place, a utilitarian claim that the good is maximized when the use of humans in research is permitted is well-known.

This utilitarian argument may be somewhat persuasive to the person with autism, but only somewhat. Chapter 3 detailed one of the problems that might emerge when a utilitarian ethic is cited to an autistic agent to justify actions—Mill's "ultimate sanction of utility" is not convincing to persons with autism. The internal sanction—a feeling of sympathy for fellow creatures that makes it impossible for agents to shrink from their responsibilities to maximize utility—is not fully operative in the person who lacks a theory of mind. The social disengagement that characterizes autism renders the ultimate sanction an ineffective motivator. Without this motivation, utilitarianism is not as persuasive, and thus the utilitarian argument for the use of human research subjects is not well-motivated either. A second concern about the applicability of the utilitarian argument addresses whether it genuinely maximizes the interests of adults with autism to participate in medical research that may hold out some type of "therapeutic" benefit. The details of this argument are laid out in the next section of the chapter.

A second argument often cited in favor of the use of human research subjects is one that makes use of Beauchamp and Childress's principles of biomedical ethics, an approach often termed "principlism." On one hand, it might be a violation of nonmaleficence to use persons as research subjects. Numerous instances have occurred in which persons were harmed by unethical research, such as research that employed unjust subject selection or inadequate (or non-existent) informed consent. However, as with any ethic of *prima facie* duties,

Beauchamp and Childress's principle of nonmaleficence should be weighed off against competing principles. The principles of justice and beneficence present justification for the use of human research subjects, so that new discoveries might benefit others. The permissibility of human subject research is bolstered by appropriate attention to the principle of autonomy, which demands that the protections of informed consent be afforded research subjects, except in the most outstanding cases. Even vulnerable subject populations, such as children or persons with mental disabilities that may affect decision making capacity, may be used as research subjects on the basis of the principle of justice, lest a failure to do so renders them therapeutic orphans.

With respect to the autistic population, however, two concerns arise with respect to the principlist argument. First, given the discussion in chapter 3, it is not clear that an ethic of *prima facie* duties is workable or persuasive to persons with autism. Second, as discussed below, the argument from the principle of justice proceeds from an assumption that it is of benefit to the cohorts of research subjects that the condition under study is investigated and ameliorated. This is the assumption that puts the "therapeutic" in "therapeutic orphan." But as argued in detail below, both the "cohort" claim and the "therapy" claim may be premature.

One familiar argument against using persons in medical research follows from the Kantian imperative to never use a human being merely as a means. Kant asserts that rational beings, such as humans, are objective ends, as opposed to subjective ends with a price. Objective ends must be treated as ends in themselves, whereas subjective ends may be used by others, and may be treated as a means to an end. This insight is the basis for Kant's formulation of the categorical imperative which states that no agent should use any rational being, whether himself or any other, merely as a means. Instead, all rational beings should be treated as ends in themselves. Given this, it would appear that using any human as a research subject is not morally permissible.

However, as discussed in chapter 3, this formulation of Kant's categorical imperative is not applicable to the person with autism. A formulation that requires agents to treat others as ends in themselves, and not merely as a means to an end, requires all agents to regard others, as well as themselves, in a particular way. Other agents should be regarded as individuals with interests, goals, and attitudes that are distinct from the goals that we have for ourselves. The autistic individual, in virtue of theory of mind deficits, may fail to recognize others as such.

The point here is *not* that inapplicability of Kantian deontology makes it permissible to treat persons with autism in whichever way the non-autistic agent chooses. The fact that Kantian deontology is not persuasive to the autistic individual is not a reason for the non-autistic person to reject Kant's position; there may be plenty of reasons to reject Kant without invoking autistic agents. Rather, the point is that the autistic agent himself may not be persuaded by the Kantian position that there is anything wrong with using persons merely as a means.

It is possible to interpret the Kantian argument as an argument for the permissibility of human subjects research, but only when that research is carried out with the protections of informed consent, clinical equipoise, and other familiar ethical protections. Kant never said that it is impermissible to *use any rational being at all;* rather, it is impermissible to use a rational being merely as a means. What it means to use someone merely as a means is a vexed question. Informed consent, for example, may be a safeguard that allows an individual to not be used merely as a means, but instead to be treated also as an end, even as he is used as a research subject. Does the inapplicability of the Kantian imperative demonstrate that persons with autism will not find informed consent a useful or appropriate safeguard? Possibly, insofar as offering informed consent is problematic in the context of theory of mind deficits. This is but one more instance of persons with autism and those without autism talking past each other about ethical concerns, as demonstrated in chapter 3.

In summary, both of the most familiar arguments for the use of human research subjects and one of the most familiar against this practice are not persuasive to autistic individuals. Even when Kantian arguments are cited as justifications for human subjects research, but only within the context of ethical safeguards like informed consent, the persuasiveness of the Kantian imperative may be lost on the person with autism.

While these arguments may not hold much sway for autistic persons, it is unlikely that these arguments will deter biomedical research on persons with autism. What is most likely is that this research will proceed within the apparatus of informed consent, a favorable balance of risks to potential benefits, and other ethical protections that the non-autistic population has come to employ. The challenge of appropriate proxy informed consent on behalf of incompetent autistic persons is a final demonstration of the ethical gulf between the autistic and non-autistic population.

Autism and Competency to Consent to Research

Informed consent is one of the cornerstones of human subject research protections. Except in extraordinary circumstances, competent individuals should always offer informed consent prior to participating in research.[3] Some persons with autism may be competent to offer informed consent to participate in research studies, and in such cases, no research should go forward without their consent. Competency is best understood as decision-relative (Buchanan and Brock 1990): an agent may be in a position to consent to some minimal risk research, but may not be in a position to consent to higher-risk research. Similarly, an agent may be in a position to judge whether to participate in a comparatively simple research protocol, but not in a position to assess whether participation in a more complex protocol is in his best interest.

Celia B. Fisher's examination of research on persons with mental retardation and developmental disabilities offers one perspective on informed consent from persons whose competency is often called into question (Fisher 2003). Fisher calls for a "goodness-of-fit" ethic of informed consent which, rather than concentrating on the deficiencies of potential research subjects, looks instead to "an examination of those aspects of the consent setting that are creating or exacerbating consent vulnerability" as well as a "consideration of how the setting can be modified to produce a consent process that best reflects and protects the consumer's hopes, values, concerns, and welfare" (Fisher 2003, 29). Fisher is correct: given that there is no one-size-fits-all assessment of competency across a given cognitive disability, researchers should do everything in their power to create an informed consent process that is as inclusive as possible. Inclusivity demands that each subject is presumed to be competent and given an opportunity to consent. Modifications to both the consent process and the research protocols should be made when appropriate by the researchers to ensure that this happens. In describing her goodness-of-fit ethic as "relational," however, Fisher occasionally equivocates between the *relational* aspect of a person's competencies and the informed consent setting, and the *relational* aspect of one person to other persons. The former sense of "relational" holds important lesson when asking persons with autism to participate in research. When vulnerable subject populations, such as persons with cognitive disabilities that affect decision making capacity, are used as research subjects, researchers should consider the competencies that the individual subject *does* have and tailor informed consent, and in some cases the research itself, so as to best allow the subject to consent to the research process. When using the latter sense of "relational," however, Fisher's claims are not as easily applicable to the person with theory of mind deficiencies:

> Adults with mental retardation, like all persons, are linked to others in relationships of reciprocity and dependency. A relational ethic calls for scientists to construct informed consent procedures based upon moral principles of respect, care, and justice guided by responsiveness to the abilities, values, and concerns of research participants and awareness of the scientists' own competencies and obligations. (Fisher 2003, 29)

> Within a relational framework autonomy need not be conceptualized as isolated or isolating, but as an expression of connectedness to others. From this perspective, when efforts to create a goodness-of-fit between the person and consent context are insufficient to insure adequate consent, individuals with mental retardation should be encouraged to select a consent partner or to yield decision-making to a consent surrogate who can help them arrive at a decision best fitting the prospective participant's wishes and concerns. (Fisher 2003, 30)

The goodness-of-fit ethic makes use of the fact that people are intimately related to other people, and these relations are the basis of an ethic of both care and justice. As seen in chapter 3, moral theories, such as Hume's, that take claims about connectedness as a basis for moral obligations stumble in the face of theory of mind deficits. It is possible that Fisher's claims about dependency and connectedness are only construed as one-way relationships, akin to the relationships that characterize Glüer and Pagin's parasitic language users. This is unlikely, however. The relationships Fisher is discussing are characterized by greater reciprocity than the mere parasitic relationships, and involve the very reciprocity that may be beyond persons with theory of mind deficiencies. Fisher's conclusions are correct. Some of her claims about the reciprocity that characterizes human relationships, and its implications for informed consent, however, do not apply to the person with autism who has an impaired theory of mind.

Fisher's conclusions force a rethinking of the notion of "competency." In their discussion of competency to consent to medical treatments, Allen E. Buchanan and Dan W. Brock distinguish two types of capacities that are necessary in order for an individual to be competent.[4] The first type is the capacity for understanding and communication, and the second type is the capacity for reasoning and deliberation (Buchanan and Brock 1990, 23). The latter are not necessarily problematic for persons with autism. Assessments of reasoning and deliberation should be made on a case-by-case basis, and there is nothing about autism that necessitates that persons with autism will be burdened by these requirements, as long as they are not required to reason or deliberate about others' complex mental states. Autism has interesting implications with respect to the former, however.

According to the DSM-IV criteria, autism is characterized by difficulties in communication (American Psychiatric Association 1994). Even for high-functioning individuals who have strong language skills, some problems in communication may persist. While Gricean and Davidsonian meaning theories are not the only meaning theories available, the difficulties that emerge for these meaning theories, in light of theory of mind deficits, may cast doubt on the communication ability of some persons with autism. More problematic than communication difficulties, however, is the capacity for understanding cited by Buchanan and Brock. They elaborate on what is required for this capacity:

> Understanding is not a merely formal or abstract process, but also requires the ability to appreciate the nature and meaning of potential alternatives—what it would be like and "feel" like to be in possible future states and to undergo various experiences—and to integrate this appreciation into one's decision making. In young children this is often prevented by the lack of sufficient life experience. In the case of elderly persons facing diseases with progressive and extremely debilitating deterioration, it is hindered by people's generally limited ability to understand a kind of experience radically different from their own, and by the inability of severely impaired individuals to communicate the character of their own experience to others. (Buchanan and Brock 1990, 24)

Buchanan and Brock are correct—understanding is an essential part of competency to consent; understanding should integrate not only rationality and abstraction, but also an appreciation of alternatives. To understand what it is to consent to a particular course of action is to understand what would happen if that action were not performed. But as discussed in chapter 1, two difficulties emerge when applying this notion of "understanding" to persons with autism. First, as illustrated by the simulation theory (ST) and theory theory (TT) debate, the abstraction that is required to employ counterfactuals that capture "a kind of experience radically different from their own" may be difficult for persons with autism. ST and TT present alternative conceptions of how behaviors by intentional agents are explained. ST avoids direct ascriptions of intentional states, and instead requires agents to merely simulate what they would do in a particular situation. TT requires agents to ascribe intentions to others when explaining their behaviors. Autism does not give definitive evidence as to which of these two theories is correct, in part because both ST and TT are both problematic for persons with autism. TT is most immediately problematic, given the direct intentional ascriptions required. But as argued in both chapters 1 and 3, ST also presents challenges, given the difficulties that persons with autism face with imaginative play, and with the appreciation of others' beliefs and preferences that are distinct from their own as characterized in the unified consciousness view. The "ability to appreciate the nature and meaning of potential alternatives" inherent in Buchanan and Brock's notion of understanding requires the same capacities as a successful employment of ST. There is little wonder that persons with autism will demonstrate what Buchanan and Brock call "generally limited ability to understand a kind of experience radically different from their own."

A second difficulty that emerges when considering Buchanan and Brock's conception of "understanding" emerges from the significance of self-awareness to understanding. If Frith and Happé are correct about the unique nature of self-consciousness in persons with autism, then communicating the character of one's own experiences to others may also be problematic for persons with autism. The difficulty is not a problem with communication per se; rather, given Frith and Happé's points about self-reflection and autism, persons with autism may not know the character of their own experiences well enough to be able to communicate them to others. *This is not to say that by definition all persons with autism are not competent decision makers.* Rather, the unique deficits that characterize autism may require researchers to be particularly careful when seeking informed consent from persons with autism in line with Fisher's recommendations. Knowledge of the difficulties that persons with autism face is necessary in order to treat persons with autism with the respect they deserve. Patience, understanding, and novel approaches to informed consent are required when obtaining consent from individuals who may have enormous difficulty in understanding alternative courses of action, or accessing their own values and preferences.

Substituted Judgments, Best Interests, Missing Cohorts

What of persons with autism who are not competent to make the decision to participate in biomedical research? When a person is not able to make medical decisions on his own behalf a proxy decision maker is asked to make decisions for that person. An affirmative decision by a proxy decision maker, or surrogate, based on an understanding of the information presented carries justificatory power making it permissible to perform an intervention on another person, even without that person's own consent. There are two standards by which surrogates can make medical decisions on behalf of those who are unable to consent. According to the first, the substituted judgment standard, surrogates make decisions for another agent based upon that agent's prior beliefs and preferences. If an agent would have consented to a particular course of action, then that is what the surrogate should consent to on that agent's behalf. Thus, the surrogate substitutes his judgment for that of the agent on behalf of whom he offers consent according to the incapacitated agent's own prior beliefs and preferences. In this sense, a surrogate is not necessarily a legally authorized representative, but one who has sufficient moral authority on the basis of knowing another's beliefs and preferences to speak on that person's behalf.

Since substituted judgments require the proxy decision maker to know the beliefs and preferences of the person for whom the surrogate is offering consent, close family member and friends are often the best surrogates. The substituted judgment standard is not applicable in certain emergent situations if no one is immediately available who knows the beliefs and preferences of the person who is not able to offer consent themselves. Nor are substituted judgments applicable for persons who were never competent to make decisions on their own behalf, such as very young children. But for individuals who were formerly competent to make decisions, but who are not able to do so at the present time, or are no longer able to do so, a substituted judgment standard is appropriate. The substituted judgment standard, however, is not applicable for those who can decide for themselves to participate in medical research; in such cases, persons should always be permitted to offer their own consent, rather than have a surrogate speak on their behalf. Autism is unlike progressively worsening conditions such as Alzheimer's—if a person with autism is not presently competent owing to autism, it is not the case that there was a time in the past during which the person was competent. Thus, the substituted judgment standard is not an appropriate means by which decisions can be made to participate in research for incompetent autistic persons. Another standard for surrogate decision making needs to be explored.

A second standard by which decisions can be made on behalf of those unable to consent for themselves is the best interest standard. According to this standard, surrogates make decisions based upon what is in the best interest of the individual on behalf of whom consent is offered. If the medical intervention under consideration is in the best interest of the incompetent person, then this fact can be cited by the proxy decision maker as a reason for consenting to the procedure. The fact that the intervention is expected to be in that person's best interest has justificatory power, allowing a medical intervention even when the person who is the object of that intervention cannot consent. Unlike the substituted judgment standard, the best interest standard does not require that proxy decision makers cite, or even know, the beliefs and preferences of the individuals for whom they offer consent. As such, the best interest standard is available to healthcare providers who do not know the beliefs and preferences of the individual, such as persons who present in emergent circumstances. This point is what motivated Veatch, in chapter 3, to examine questions about what makes for a good life for human beings. Decisions made on behalf of very young children, or persons born with cognitive disabilities which affect decision making ability, can be made using a best interest standard. Thus, the best interest standard would appear to be a basis for proxy decision makers to make decisions on behalf of persons with autism who are not presently, nor ever were, competent to make medical decisions on their own.

Strikingly, however, an argument exists that demonstrates that the participation of adults with autism in some biomedical experiments *cannot* be justified using a best interest standard. This argument is limited in scope to adults with autism, and those medical studies that investigate potential cures for autism, such as remedies for theory of mind deficits. The argument is not applicable to research studies that are designed to investigate the nature of autism in non-invasive ways, such that there is no possibility that the experiment might "cure" autism in the research subjects. So, for example, the Sally-Anne or Smarties tasks described in chapter 1 do not fall under the scope of the argument presented below. Biomedical, as opposed to behavioral studies, which are more invasive, and which are designed to directly address theory of mind deficits, are the focus of the argument.

The argument proceeds from the uncontroversial description of the best interest standard: it is appropriately invoked when the intervention in question is believed to be in the best interest of the person on behalf of whom consent is offered. The unique way in which theory of mind deficits shape who a person with autism is has stunning repercussions for the application of the best interest standard:

(1) If biomedical research on persons with autism who have always been incompetent to consent to participate in research can appropriately be consented to on the basis of a best interest standard, then participating in biomedical research is in the best interest of the autistic research subject;

(2) Participating in non-therapeutic biomedical research is not in the best interest of autistic research subjects;

(3) Participating in therapeutic biomedical research is not in the best interest of autistic research subjects;

(4) Therefore, from (2) and (3), there is no biomedical research in which autistic research subjects can participate that is in their best interest;

(5) Therefore, from (1) and (4), biomedical research on persons with autism who have always been incompetent to consent to participate in research cannot be consented to on the basis of a best interest standard.

Understanding the above argument requires an examination of therapeutic and non-therapeutic research. While the designation between therapeutic and non-therapeutic research has been contested, in this context "therapeutic research" refers to research that may result in the partial or total restoration of theory of mind, and "non-therapeutic research" refers to research into the etiology of autism that does not present the possibility of restoring theory of mind.

While all human subjects research must result in greater net benefit than net risks, benefits can accrue in one of two ways. In some cases, benefits accrue directly to the subjects themselves, although future patients may also benefit from the knowledge gained from the study. Medical research that may directly benefit subjects is considered therapeutic research. However, there are some cases in which benefits are not expected to accrue directly to the subjects in the research. Perhaps a new drug is being introduced into a population to study if the drug can be tolerated by that population, but not to test for benefits to the subjects per se. The drug may ultimately benefit the population in which the drug is initially tested, but the study was not designed with this expectation. In such cases, the benefits are *aspirational*—the benefit in performing the research may accrue to future patients, but not to the subjects themselves (King 2000). Research in which the benefits are solely aspirational is non-therapeutic research—research that is not expected to have any therapeutic benefit to the subject himself. While benefits may be either direct or aspirational, the risks of research do not divide along these lines. Even though the benefits may accrue either to the subjects of the study, or to future patients, in all biomedical research the risks of the research are borne primarily by the subjects.[5] In summary, (1) the benefits of research may be either direct, as in the case of therapeutic research, or aspirational, as in the case of non-therapeutic research; (2) the risks of research are shouldered almost exclusively by the subjects themselves; and finally, (3) as long as the net benefits, be they direct or aspirational, outweigh the risks, the requirement for a positive risk/benefit ratio is fulfilled.

Therapeutic research is typically considered less controversial than research that results in only aspirational, not direct, benefits.[6] Why is therapeutic research less controversial? One reason stems from the implicit assumption that even with full and voluntary informed consent some measure of autonomy is compromised by virtue of being a research subject. Perhaps the very condition that qualifies a person as a research subject for most biomedical research is one that inherently compromises autonomy. For example, the only way to successfully assess the therapeutic benefits of a new cancer treatment is to test it on patients with cancer. If having cancer results in some internal constraint on the part of the subject, then the very condition that qualifies her as a subject is one that compromises her autonomy. A second reason that therapeutic research is considered less controversial is that even if a subject does not view the condition that qualifies her as a subject as one that is inherently autonomy-limiting, being a research subject may nonetheless be autonomy-limiting in itself. Research subjects are asked to take on medical regimens that they otherwise would not accept, on schedules that may not be to their liking, and undergo tests to which they might not otherwise accede. However, the trade-off in participating in potentially therapeutic research may outweigh the loss of autonomy. Some autonomy is lost, but some other benefit may be gained, thereby negating some of the ills of a loss of autonomy. For these reasons, non-therapeutic research, which does not confer the possibility of direct benefit to outweigh the loss of autonomy faced by the subject, is judged more ethically problematic. The Declaration of Helsinki sets out additional provisions for non-therapeutic research, precisely because of this assumption that non-therapeutic research may be more ethically problematic than therapeutic research (World Medical Association 2004). Sections 46.406–407 of the Common Rule make clear that research on children which carries greater than minimal risk but which is not expected to benefit those children directly must meet the highest of standards before it may be approved (Department of Health and Human Services 2005). The term "therapeutic misconception" was coined precisely because the errant assumption that non-therapeutic research might confer some benefit is rampant among potential subjects, and because this errant assumption could place individuals in morally compromising positions (Appelbaum et al. 1987). One consequence of the therapeutic misconception is that individuals may agree to participate in research which is not expected to benefit them directly, trading in their autonomy for little, if any, direct benefit.

The assumption behind the claim that non-therapeutic research is more ethically problematic than therapeutic research is the assumption that *it is of benefit to people with a condition under study to be cured of that condition*. Research that results in therapy is directly beneficial, whereas non-therapeutic research that results in mere aspirational benefits is a distant second choice. This discussion of therapeutic and non-therapeutic research sets the stage to return to the argument about the applicability of the best interest standard as a standard of surrogate consent for persons with autism. The first premise of this argument merely sets out a basic requirement of the best interest standard. The best interest standard is only applicable when it is genuinely in the best interest of the person on behalf of whom consent is offered to participate in the biomedical experiment.

The second premise is uncontroversial: non-therapeutic biomedical experiments are not in the best interest of research subjects. That is why the standards are so high for permitting such research, and why the Common Rule demands research on children which exceeds minimal risk and which is expected to not have any direct benefit for those children meet the highest level of ethical scrutiny. Research into the causes of autism or the nature of autism, such as false-belief tasks, may not benefit the person who participates in that research directly, although there may be some benefits to participation that do not accrue directly as a result of the experimental intervention. Participation may qualify individuals for free medical services, or a cash incentive. In this sense, participation may be of some "benefit" to the autistic participant, although not of therapeutic benefit. Such benefits are themselves ethically questionable, and can be seen as coercive. The fact that cash payments, for example, may be coercive to the most autonomous of potential research subjects demonstrates that, *a fortiori*, they would be coercive to incompetent research subjects. But when it comes to invasive biomedical experiments, the nature of non-therapeutic research is that the individual research subjects bear the burden of risk, without expectation of direct benefit from participation in the study.

The most controversial premise is premise three. If the research is not merely an investigation of the causes or nature of autism, or behavioral aspects of autism, but research on adults into a potential "cure" for autism, with the possibility of this cure as one of the therapeutic benefits, the question emerges as to whether this is of benefit to the subject at all. It is the case that future persons are benefited by not being born with autism. In chapter 2, arguments established that part of what it is to lead a full human life is to enter into reciprocal relationships of the kind not available to persons without a theory of mind. It would be better for future children that they are not born with autism. It is not as clear that adults who have always lacked theory of mind would be benefited by gaining theory of mind in mid-life: who they are would be compromised tremendously by gaining theory of mind. Therapeutic research designed to benefit them may not be a benefit to autistic adults at all.

It may be jarring to move from a world in which full intentionality is not ascribed to other humans into a world in which others suddenly are rendered more complex. The full degree of the challenge in moving from the autistic world into the non-autistic world may not be fully appreciated, because individuals who are not autistic cannot imagine what it would be like to move from the autistic world into the non-autistic world. While it would be difficult for the autistic person with a newly acquired theory of mind to come to grips with the complexity of other persons, it would be just as difficult to come to grips with the complexity of *oneself* with a newly acquired theory of mind. In chapter 1, the repercussions for self-consciousness of a compromised theory of mind were laid out. It is not merely a newfound understanding of others that the formerly autistic person would have to accept, but a new understanding of the self. Being "cured" of autism requires a person to undergo radical reconsideration of not only other persons, but also himself. If this is not of direct benefit to him, there is similarly no reason to expect that there are aspirational benefits to be gained from this research, allowing future adults with autism to be "cured."

Lines four and five follow from the previously established premises. The surprising conclusion is that the best interest standard is not applicable to some types of biomedical research on persons with autism. In particular, the best interest standard cannot be used to offer ethical justification for the use of adults with autism for research studies that have the therapeutic benefit of possibly restoring the subject's theory of mind.

The objections to this argument focus on the most controversial premise, premise three. One objection revisits the distinction between three theories of the good discussed by Scanlon, Veatch, and Parfit in chapter 2. The first of these theories is an experiential theory, or hedonistic theory—what is good for a person is what gives him pleasure. The second is a desire theory—what is good for a person is what fulfills his or her desires. The third theory is an objective list theory—what is good for a person are those things that are found on a list of objective goods for human beings, including relationships with other human beings. Persons with theory of mind deficits are missing out on one of the goods on the objective lists, and while it may be jarring to be "cured" of autism, the fact that they are now able to appreciate all of the goods on the objective list must surely be good for them. This position is in keeping with Nussbaum's points about human capabilities. There are some capabilities that persons with autism do not have. Surely it is best to restore these capabilities and to do what we can in order to restore them for anyone who currently fails to have them. Thus, this research really is therapeutic, and being cured of autism really would be of benefit to the person with autism.

The appeal to the objective lists is mistaken, however. Parfit's lesson, that experiential theories and objective list theories must complement each other, is instructive here. Chapter 2 made reference to Parfit's observation that the goods of the objective list are not that good if an agent does not receive pleasure from them; thus the experiential and objective list theories go hand in hand. This may account for Scanlon's and others' failure to develop objective lists in too much detail—each individual may derive pleasure from each of the items on the objective list to a slightly different degree, or in a different fashion. There is no one-size-fits-all objective list, even if there is widespread agreement on many of the components of the objective lists. To return to the adult with autism: after years of not receiving pleasure from some of the items on the non-autistic objective list, can an adult with autism be suddenly expected to welcome the deluge of reciprocal relationships that characterize the non-autistic objective lists? The flip side of this is the mistaken assumption that the person with autism was not receiving pleasure from the items on his own list, such as bus schedules, prime numbers, or antique watches. The pleasures of folk physics are not substitutes for, but they are just as real as, the pleasures of folk psychology. To hastily conclude that any person would welcome a new set of items on his objective list, and eschew those items that have long given him pleasure, is to fail to recognize that individual as an individual. Adults *without* autism have distinct beliefs and preferences, such that you cannot in mid-life expect them to suddenly welcome a new way of looking at the world, or looking at themselves. Adults *with* autism should not be expected to be any different. Any suggestion of re-making the world of an adult with autism—an adult with his own personality, beliefs, and preferences—is a failure to recognize him as his own person.

Another objection is that the argument proves too much. The argument appears to support the untenable position that there is no therapeutic research that is morally acceptable. Substitute "cancer" or "blindness" for "autism" in the above argument, this objection states, and the argument shows exactly that. Any argument that concludes cancer or blindness should not be researched is mistaken, as the therapeutic benefits of such research are clearly warranted. Is the same true of autism? Those who make this argument have not paid sufficient attention to the uniqueness of autism. Autism does not merely change the way that individuals interact with the world—it changes the very nature of the self, and the very nature of the other inhabitants of the world with whom the autistic person interacts. Blindness restricts the nature of communication with other persons, but it does not challenge a blind person's abilities to interact with other persons *qua* persons. Narratives of illness are replete with descriptions of the ways in which cancer changes the relationship that people have with themselves, and with others. But the poignancy that characterizes these narratives results from the pain that can emerge from loneliness, isolation, or loss of relationships with others. The uniqueness of autism is that the pain in the loneliness, isolation, or loss of relationships is not necessarily as great, and in some cases, is not there at all.

Perhaps in this sense autism is akin to schizophrenia, a disorder that radically changes a person's view of reality or of himself. But autism is different even from that, for three reasons. First, people are not born schizophrenic; they develop the condition, and in most cases, comparatively late in life. Even those rare cases of childhood-onset schizophrenia occur, in most cases, late enough that "linguistic and cognitive development is substantially completed" (Frith 2003, 69). Persons with schizophrenia come to know the nature of the self and others before their understanding is compromised by their illness. In the case of autism, however, people are either born with the condition, or if they have a regressive form, begin to evidence autistic traits as very young children. Unlike persons with schizophrenia, adults with autism have never experienced any other way of being. Second, there are drugs that can be used to treat many of the symptoms of schizophrenia, many of which work well. Coupled with the later-onset claim above, the fact that drugs exist that treat many symptoms of schizophrenia creates the possibility that persons with schizophrenia may maintain the relationships with the self and others that they had prior to the onset of the disease. This is actually the weakest of the three points, as there is nothing in principle that would prevent the development of therapies that might treat some of the distressing symptoms of autism, such as sensory difficulties. Third, and most significantly, autism is characterized by theory of mind deficits, which compromise the person with autism's ability to interact with other persons *qua* persons. As seen in chapter 2, this is part of what makes a human life a *human* life, a life worth living. The person with schizophrenia may make certain mistakes about the people around her—she may think them untrustworthy or inconsistent—but she has no doubt that there are *intentional agents* around her with whom she can richly interact. Theory of mind deficits cut off an essential component of this interaction.

An additional objection to the argument disputes premise two, arguing that the aspirational benefits of non-therapeutic research are given short shrift. Non-therapeutic research may not be of direct benefit to the subjects, but it may contribute to knowledge about autism. This research may benefit others with autism—the cohort of research subjects with autism—a goal that many persons with autism may wish to fulfill. Barry Brown's cohort interest argument attempts to forge a narrow ground between the wide-ranging good sought by the utilitarian argument for human subjects research, and research that is expected to promote only aspirational benefits. And yet, even Brown's attempt to split the difference comes up short when considering autistic research subjects.

Brown considers the ethical quandary posed by individuals who cannot consent to participate in research, such as elderly patients with Alzheimer's disease. What can justify the use of persons with severe dementia in biomedical research, especially research that is not expected to be of direct benefit to subjects themselves? Brown envisions that individuals who cannot consent to research may nonetheless have surrogates who make decisions based on the substituted judgment that individuals have an interest in promoting the good for their community. The decision to enroll a patient with advanced dementia, for example, as a research subject "is justified by the claim, if valid, that it is for the common good of the dementia-care-research community, of which he is a member and to which, it is presumed, he would commit himself if he were capable of doing so at the time" (Brown 2006, 244). A community of patients exists, comprised of individuals who "have, even if they have never explicitly associated with each other, common values and disvalues" (Brown 2006, 243), and who would not wish for their friends or relatives to have the same condition that befell them. The formerly competent research subject may not have explicitly agreed to participate in research. She may not have had explicit beliefs or preferences about this while still competent, because at that time she did not have the illness that is being studied. The research subject who was never competent would not have had beliefs and preferences about participating in these research studies. However, both populations share an affinity with the community of persons who do have this disorder. Thus, even research subjects who are not competent would wish for their cohorts to be benefited by their own participation in medical studies.

It is clear that Brown's cohort interest argument is not sufficient to demonstrate the falsity of premise three. As discussed in chapter 4, it is a misnomer to speak of the Autistic community, in the sense that there are persons with autism who share values, beliefs, and interests with other persons who have autism. There is an Autistic community comprised overwhelmingly of persons *without* autism who advocate on behalf of those persons with autism, but their interests alone are not sufficient for the cohort interest argument to go through. It would not be ethical to claim that research on an incompetent subject is justified on the basis of the fact that some community, of whom that subject never considered himself or would never consider himself a member, nonetheless has an interest in that person's participation in the research. Such a claim treads too closely to a justification of human subjects research on the basis of unchecked act-utilitarianism, which as mentioned above, cannot be invoked to justify human subjects research.

At this point one of the central mysteries of autism, sensory difficulties, emerges to further confound the argument. It has been hypothesized that theory of mind difficulties are casually connected to sensory difficulties. One version of this hypothesis is called the salience landscape theory (Ramachandran and Oberman 2006). According to this theory, the connections between the amygdala, which determines appropriate emotional responses to sensory stimuli, and the sensors themselves is disrupted in persons with autism. The result is that the autistic person's salience landscape is not what it should be, rendering bright lights, high-pitched sounds, or scratchy clothing nearly unbearable. A second hypothesis postulates that extreme aversion to touch, or the over-stimulating experience of eye contact, causes infants with autism to push away from other people. The result is that these infants never learn the basics of theory of mind, precisely because sensory over-stimulation drives a wedge between them and other people early in life. If the second version of the sensory difficulties hypothesis is true, then perhaps research designed to ameliorate sensory difficulties might result in curing theory of mind deficits. Once touch or eye contact is no longer painful, perhaps a person with theory of mind deficits might find his or her own way back to a world of reciprocal relationships. This is not likely, for two reasons. First, it may be argued that the acquisition of theory of mind is something that can only be achieved in childhood. Fluency in theory of mind, like fluency in a foreign language, may only be mastered when one is exposed from a very young age. Once someone is an adult, the window is closed. There is a second, more significant objection to this theory, however. It is question-begging. If eye contact is too stimulating, it must be so precisely because the person who finds it too stimulating recognizes that there is a mind behind those eyes. Looking into another human's eyes is not the same as looking at a picture of human eyes. But for one pair to be too stimulating, and the other to not be, is not merely because one is in three dimensions, and the other is a two-dimensional representation. Rather, it is because of the recognition that there is a mind behind the eyes in one case, eyes that are scrutinizing the observer in a particular way. But if that is true, then the sensory overload that results from eye contact is predicated on the recognition of others' mental states. It makes no sense to say that a *lack of theory of mind* is caused by stimulation that is unbearable *because of theory of mind*. Thus, the hypothesis that theory of mind is caused by sensory over-stimulation is not plausible.

Ramachandran and Oberman's salience landscape theory remains intact in the face of this objection, however. With it comes the ethical question: should research on persons with autism who are unable to consent to research be permitted for research designed to remedy sensory difficulties? As stated earlier in this chapter, the results of these treatments might be akin to wearing sunglasses, restricting light on one hand, but allowing greater visibility on the other. Especially in cases where sensory overload is causing a person with autism pain, it is clear that such research is of therapeutic benefit to the autistic research participant himself, as well as to future persons with autism. Thus, such research is morally permissible.

While the above discussion considers the complexities in using adults with autism as research subjects in biomedical studies that may remedy theory of mind deficits, the argument does not apply to children with autism. Donna Chen et al. observe that a considerable amount of research on autism will be on very young children (Chen et al. 2003, 49). In the case of young children, it is possible that their view of other persons as well as their own self-concept is not solidified, such that the acquisition of theory of mind would not prove to be harmful. Instead, the early acquisition of theory of mind would allow a child to ultimately experience the full range of Nussbaum's human capabilities, or the constituents of Scanlon's, Veatch's, and Parfit's conceptions of well-being. Thus, research that may remedy theory of mind deficits in children is morally acceptable.

With respect to this type of research, however, the possibility of the therapeutic misconception emerges. Parents may have outsized expectations about the therapeutic benefits of research on children with autism. In such cases, it is imperative that researchers are as clear as possible about the expected value of the research. One recommendation that is often made to researchers who are working with a vulnerable population group, such as persons with dementia or other cognitive disabilities that may affect decision making capacity, is that the researchers take each interaction with their subjects as an opportunity to reiterate informed consent. Parents of children with autism may not be subjects of the research themselves, but they are the ones who offer consent on behalf of their children, and in virtue of having a child with autism they are vulnerable. Researchers should take each interaction with such parents to reiterate the limits of the expected benefits of their study so that parents do not labor under a therapeutic misconception.

In summary, it is not necessarily of benefit for adults with autism to participate in research studies that may hold out the possibility of a "cure" for autism. Children with autism may yet be able to acquire theory of mind without forcing them to radically re-think their notion of others, as well as re-think their notion of the self. But rather than involving adults with autism in biomedical experiments that might drastically change their relationships with others, and change their understanding of the self, adults with autism should be allowed to live out the lives the way they are. Respect for a life without theory of mind, and a notion of autistic integrity, is called for.

An Ethic of Autistic Integrity

We don't have a disease, so we can't be "cured." This is just the way we are.

JACK THOMAS, A 10TH GRADER AT A SCHOOL FOR AUTISTIC TEENAGERS (HARMON 2004)

Autistic integrity recognizes that adults with autism see other people, and themselves, differently than the non-autistic population; further-more, this is the only way that they know how to be. Jack Thomas may be overstating the case in saying that autism is not a disease, but he is correct in saying that for autistic adults this *is* just the way that they are. Two points should be made in reference to autistic integrity. First, while theory of mind deficits persist, many adults with autism learn how to compensate for these deficits. Some adults with autism can compensate for a lack of theory of mind (Frith 2003). This is not to say that they are able to acquire theory of mind late in life. Rather, they learn to navigate the world without theory of mind. This is not the same as having a full understanding of "mentalese," but it is still possible to have a full and engaging life without theory of mind. Those people with autism who do come to have an explicit theory of mind may do so via their own process and on their own terms. The process can in some cases be quite difficult, and can take place over a long period of time (Frith and Happé 1999). They can recognize others in the fullest sense. The call for autistic integrity concerns those persons with autism who cannot recognize others in the fullest sense, however.

The second aspect of autistic integrity recognizes that changing an autistic person into someone who has a theory of mind would require him to undergo a fundamental shift in the way that he interacts with others and understands himself. In promoting "autistic integrity" it is important not to romanticize persons with autism, or autism itself.[7] Rather, the focus should be on recognizing that persons with autism may lack theory of mind, cutting them off in significant ways from other people, but for adults with autism, this is the only way that they know how to be. Among the lessons of Frith and Happé's work on autism and self-consciousness is that people without autism do not know what it would be like to be autistic; similarly, those with autism do not know what it would be like to not be autistic. The way that we come to understand each other's actions is different; what our self-consciousness consists of may be different; what we mean when we use words is different; what counts as a good life for us is different; and the theories available to us to determine what is morally right and wrong are different. Parents are justified in performing actions in order to prevent their future children from being autistic, because so much of what non-autistic parents recognize as the constituents of an objectively good life are missing for persons who are autistic. For adults with autism, however, these considerations come too late.

One last attempt might be offered: is it not wrong to not attempt to change adults with autism, who are perpetually cut off from what Scanlon, Veatch, Parfit, and Nussbaum rightly recognize as part of a well-lived human life? Even if Parfit is correct that an objective list without pleasure is empty and unfulfilling, once an adult with autism has the opportunity to engage in reciprocal relationships, surely he will come to take pleasure in them. Once theory of mind is restored, then the pleasure inherent in reciprocal relationships will come. So too will a renewed sense of the self, one that is so much richer than that which persons with autism currently experience.

The problem with this position is that it fails to recognize that persons with autism are individuals, with personalities and preferences just as varied as those of the non-autistic population. It is a similar moral wrong to the one discussed in chapter 3, which postulated that persons with autism should be valued because they make non-autistic people better. That claim was demonstrated to be false: saying that autistic persons are valuable because of what they offer the non-autistic population fails to value autistic persons for themselves. Similarly, to foist a "cure" on a person with autism fails to recognize him as a person in his own right, because that cure assumes that the person would be better off cured. There is no reason to assume that once theory of mind is restored that an adult with a mature set of preferences would undergo a personality shift such that he would suddenly come to enjoy the world of mentalizing. If a member of the non-autistic population were confronted with a comparable option—"Let us change you fundamentally, and trust us, you will come to love your new life"—we would find this a horrific violation of that person's autonomy. The person's integrity as an autonomous individual would be compromised. As stated above, curing cancer or restoring sight to a person who was blind would not fundamentally change that individual *qua* person. But restoring theory of mind would.

An ethic that requires the non-autistic population to respect the differences of the autistic population places burdens on the non-autistic population. Family members may spend extensive resources to care for relatives with autism who are unable to care for themselves. Therapy that will help autistic persons to better care for themselves is certainly called for, and distributive justice demands that greater resources are spent by society to create educational opportunities. Distributive justice demands that the autistic population is served as well as possible, and once they are adults, it is wrong to try to make an autistic person into someone he is not, and someone he does not want to be. Investments to integrate persons with autism into society should be viewed as any other investment in integrating persons with disabilities into a society that often does not do enough to promote accessibility. Abigail Sullivan Moore describes a program at Keene State College in New Hampshire that provides fellow students a "social navigators" for students with Asperger's (Moore 2006). Social navigators are to persons with autism what audio books or Braille books are to persons who are blind: a way to enable persons to engage with the world. It is not the case that every child with autism will eventually go to college—just as every typically developing child does not ultimately go to college. But this program is one example of what can be done to uphold autistic integrity, and to help students who wish to go to college. At a similar program at the University of Minnesota, students are assisted in navigating the university food court and bus service. Lisa King, who works with student in the Minnesota program, asks rhetorically, "We would provide an interpreter to a hard-of-hearing person. Why don't we provide an interpreter for somebody with Asperger's?" (Moore 2006).

Happé observes that "The central coherence account of autism, then, predicts skills as well as failures, and as such can best be characterised not as a deficit account, but in terms of cognitive style" (Happé 2000, 205–206). Similarly, any account of autism that identifies the lack of theory of mind as characterizing autism must recognize that the lack of theory of mind is simply the way that some adults are. It would have been better for each autistic individual if, from birth, he or she had an intact theory of mind. That person would be able to enjoy all of the human capabilities, enter into fully reciprocal relationships, and speak the same moral language as non-autistic persons. But as an adult, each autistic person should be appreciated for who he or she is.

In April 2007 an article in the *New York Times* cited Temple Grandin and her work on humane farming practices. Here is what the author said:

> Temple Grandin, an animal science professor at Colorado State University who is a pioneer in the field of humane cattle handling, said public pressure on meat producers in the last few years has been "building and building to where I feel we're at a tipping point now."
>
> When she spoke at last week's conference on animal care at the annual American Meat Institute in Kansas City, Mo., she said, there were more than 300 people in attendance. "That's more than we've ever had before, and I think it's a wonderful sign," she said. (Vitello 2007)

There is no mention of autism in the article, which cites Grandin one additional time. Why should there be?

Notes

Introduction

1. The "problem of other minds" can be briefly summed up as the problem that we are unable to determine, with certainty, that other persons have minds. While we have direct access to our own minds, we operate on the mere assumption that other persons have minds. The behaviorist versus functionalist debate is an attempt to address this question. My working assumption throughout this book is that functionalism is true (i.e., other typically developed persons have minds which function in the same way as do our own), and that intentional explanations of human behavior—including good dashes of folk psychology—are also true. See Richard Gipps (2004) for a rejection of some of these psychological and philosophical assumptions.

2. See, for example, a discussion of this quotation's disputed provenance at the Gallaudet University website, http://library.gallaudet.edu/deaf-faq-helen-keller.shtml (accessed January 4, 2008). Librarians at Gallaudet have not been able to find the original source of the quotation, although they have twice located the same sentiment in Keller's writings.

3. See the discussion in chapter 1 for the ways in which early impediments in language acquisition on the part of deaf children initially impede theory of mind development, and the fact that eventual language competency on the part of deaf persons comes hand in hand with an understanding of theory of mind that outpaces that of persons with autism.

1. A Philosophical Introduction to Autism

1. Another thesis, that persons with autism have overselective visuospacial attention, has received less attention from philosophers (Plaisted 2000).

2. Hutto refers to the unified consciousness view as one in which a person sees the world "mono-perspectively" (Hutto 2003); Goldman calls it "egocentric biases" (Goldman 2006). One consequence of the unified consciousness view would be that autistic persons fail to have empathy for others' troubles. See chapter 3 for further discussion.

3. See Baron-Cohen (2000b) for additional theory of mind tests that do not include false belief attribution.

4. This is not to say that theory of mind deficits are themselves diagnostic. They cannot be diagnostic, because if they were, then it would be the case that persons with autism would uniquely have theory of mind deficits (the sufficient condition) and that theory of mind deficits would be universal among persons with autism (the necessary condition). Neither of these is the case. See Charman (2000) for a comprehensive discussion of the failure of theory of mind as a diagnostic tool, as well as a theory of precursors to theory of mind that anticipates Gerrans's (2002) position on the absence of a theory of mind module.

5. Victoria McGeer presents a third possibility which she terms "psycho-practical know-how" or "psycho-practical expertise," in which an understanding of others is predicated on "the internalization of normatively guided practices of mind" (McGeer 2001, 111). Shaun Gallagher presents an alternative he calls "interaction theory," comprised of two elements, *primary intersubjectivity*, the "embodied, sensory-motor (emotion-informed) capabilities that enable us to perceive the intentions of others" and *secondary intersubjectivity*, the "embodied, perceptual, and action capabilities that enable us to understand others in pragmatically contextualized situations of everyday life" (Gallagher 2004, 209).

6. See Goldman (2006) for another review of the TT versus ST debate.

7. Having defending theory theory in the past, Nichols and Stich more recently have claimed that while theory theory is still preferable to simulation theory, that "productive debate will require more detailed proposals and sharper distinctions" (Nichols and Stich, 2003, 161). For purposes of a book primarily on ethics and autism, the level of debate found here is illuminating. For those further interested in the TT versus ST debate, a more thorough discussion is available. See Stich and Nichols (1997), and Nichols and Stich (1998).

8. Barker holds that philosophical arguments alone may not be sufficient to determine which of these theories is simpler, and attempts to demonstrate the superior simplicity of ST using a computer program. The program attempts to replicate the processes by which both TT and ST would execute. See Barker (2002).

9. See also Erevelles (2002) for a discussion of the challenges "of being required to define the coherence of the 'deviant' subject according to positivist rules and humanist rationality" (Erevelles 2002, 25).

10. The question of self-consciousness has significance even if it does not bear on the TT and ST debate. It is at least possible that placing one's own propositional attitudes off-line is not a conscious endeavor; thus ST may be accomplished even without self-consciousness. Perhaps this is done automatically: without awareness of the replacement of our own propositional attitudes with those of other agents, we effortlessly and unconsciously substitute our own attitudes with those of the agents whose actions are explained using ST. While this is possible, it is not very plausible, as illustrated by examples in which agents simulate intentional states radically different from their own. When we aim to explain another agent's actions that require us to simulate intentions we find unpleasant or distasteful—If I were John, I would eat three raw eggs for breakfast; if I were John, I would close the gaping wound with my bare hands—we *are* conscious of swapping our own attitudes with those of someone else. The fact that less fantastic applications of ST occur without our conscious awareness of the attitudes that are being moved on- and

off-line is not sufficient to demonstrate that this goes on *without* conscious involvement. Rather, in normal circumstances we are just very good at simulating quickly and effortlessly. If ST is true, we would have to be that good.

11. See also Shanker (2004) who believes that the theory of mind theory of autism presupposes a Cartesian model of emotion which should be supplanted by a dynamic developmental model of emotions.

12. One question that remains unanswered concerns the relationship between theory of mind and language proficiency. Is it the case that theory of mind is necessary for proficiency in language, or does language proficiency facilitate acquisition of theory of mind? See de Villiers's review of the connections between theory of mind and language (de Villiers 2000). See also Garfield et al. (2001) for a discussion of this question, as well as their answer that "the development of language, and the development of a set of social skills are prior to, jointly causally sufficient, and individually causally necessary, for the acquisition of [theory of mind] in contradistinction both to strongly modular theories of the genesis of [theory of mind] and 'theory theory' accounts" (Garfield et al. 2001, 496). See also Tager-Flusberg and Joseph (2005) for an explanation as to how some persons with autism are able to pass theory of mind tasks, owing to their understanding of sentential complements (such as "asked," "thought," or "knew") regardless of more general language capability.

13. The non-autistic person who remembers the words by constructing a story about an *enigmatic lion who takes a harrowing ride on a greasy wheelbarrow towards a fork in the road* proves this point.

14. The point here parallels the significance of salience in particularism and the problems that this moral theory poses for persons with autism. See chapter 3.

15. Sinclair tells the story of four autistic people alone in a room who are unable to converse with each other until a non-autistic person enters the room to give "structure to the conversation" (Sinclair 1992, 299).

16. While these nine properties are classically described as the features of mental modules, there is some debate as to whether all nine are essential to mental modules. Garfield et al. (2001) argue that speed and mandatoriness are the only essential features, and they also discuss the position of Coltheart (1999) who holds that domain specificity is the sole essential property of a module.

17. Scholl and Leslie's (1999) discussion of synchronic versus diachronic modularity will be of particular appeal to those interested in varieties of modules and ways in which modules can develop.

18. Many blind or deaf children lag behind their sighted or hearing peers in initially developing a theory of mind and passing false-belief tests. This shows that shortcomings in the acquisition of mindreading concepts, and not a failure of mindreading itself, accounts for poor theory of mind competence in many cases, echoing Raffman's "Conceptual Incompetence" hypothesis. Without shared attention, such as following eye-gaze direction, or easy communication about intentional concepts, children do not perform well on false-belief tests. However, blind or deaf children eventually learn these concepts, and then perform just as well as their peers (Gerrans 2002, 317).

19. See, for example, Ponnet et al. (2005) for a discussion of high-functioning adults, some of whom had autism or Asperger's syndrome, which implicates that "under some

circumstances, some high functioning adults with PDD [pervasive developmental disorders] are able to read the thoughts and feelings of others during a naturalistic conversation" (Ponnet et al. 2005, 597). The eleven participants in their study were asked to participate in the study "on the basis of their good performance on previous mind-reading tasks" (Ponnet et al. 2005, 597). Blind or deaf children who do not have autism, but initially do poorly on false-belief tests, typically do better on other tests of theory of mind, and ultimately outpace their counterparts with autism on false-belief tests (Baron-Cohen 2000b).

20. For a discussion of the results of a study in which children with autism were able to make this distinction, see chapter 3.

2. The Value of an Autistic Life

1. See, for example, Joseph Fletcher (1972).

2. As cited by Warren, John Noonan (1968) claims that whoever is conceived of by human beings is human, and that it is morally wrong to kill humans; since fetuses are conceived of by human beings, fetuses are human, and thus killing a fetus is morally wrong.

3. This calls into question the necessary condition, but not the sufficient condition. Questions about the sufficient condition are the basis of one of the debates between Frith and Happé on one hand, and McGeer on the other, in chapter 1.

4. Nussbaum's list has changed slightly over time; she recognizes that this list may undergo further modification. For example, her 1995 list included "separateness" and "strong separateness," whereas the 2006 list eschews these for political and material control over one's environment.

5. Nussbaum acknowledges that "the area of reciprocity" is where the disabling characteristics of Asperger's syndrome manifest themselves (Nussbaum 2006, 97).

3. Autism and Moral Theories

1. For moral philosophers who are interested in Blair's moral/conventional distinction, he cites Smetana (1985) as a source for this distinction. Blair says this of the distinction: "Within the literature, moral transgressions (e.g., hitting another, damaging another's property) are defined by their consequences for the rights and welfare of others. Conventional transgressions (e.g., talking in class, dressing in opposite-sex clothes) are defined by their consequences for the social order" (Blair 1996, 572). It is notable that this is a teleological account of morality, not a deontological one. Additionally, it is one that fails to take into account "duties to the self," *per* a Kantian or Rossian system. Given both the attention to the rights of others, as well as the restriction of morality only to those actions that affect others, it is certainly not a utilitarian account. Furthermore, many cases of "talking in class" could certainly be morally wrong on utilitarian accounts, given the appropriate utilities; it is almost certainly morally wrong on Kantian and Rossian grounds. Thus, many moral philosophers may have two quibbles with Blair's study. First, the very definition of moral transgression seems to be question-begging in favor of some moral theory; and, second, the moral/conventional distinction does not appear to hold up.

2. In saying that the participants scored "at ceiling," Grant et al. (2005) were not making a claim that deontological theories were superior to consequentialist ones, but rather that the participants were consistent in their responses that arbitrarily scored consequentialist responses at one extreme and deontological ones at another.

3. The distinction between sympathy and empathy parallels Frith's distinction between instinctive empathy and intentional empathy. See Frith (2003, 111–112).

4. Kennett is concerned primarily with high-functioning persons with autism, all of whom have some theory of mind, "though [their theory of mind] may be hard won and much more laborious and explicit than the theory you and I use" (Kennett 2002, 345).

5. The contention that we are unable to keep these simulations off-line parallels the mandatoriness claims made about a theory of mind module. The ethical implications of a theory of mind deficit proceed in the absence of a definite claim about the existence of a module for theory of mind, but it is notable that Hare's observation anticipates this development.

6. The problem of an autistic individual's motivation to accept a particular moral theory is not merely a problem for utilitarianism. Kennett raises the question as to why an autistic person would choose a moral system at all. Echoing Frith and Happé, it is possible that the autistic person may lack the unity of a concept of self that is required to conceive of oneself as a moral agent (Kennett 2002, 357). If you do not conceive of yourself as an agent, why then choose a moral system? See chapter 1 for a more detailed discussion of autism and self-consciousness.

7. Interestingly, many people with autism have great difficulty deceiving others, thereby in many cases adhering to the Kantian perfect duty to others to not lie. A result of theory of mind difficulties is that persons with autism do not recognize the complexity of others' beliefs, such as the fact that others' beliefs are based on principles such as "seeing leads to knowing"; thus, deception proves difficult for them (Baron-Cohen 2000; see also chapter 1). Persons with autism may not be deceitful, but insofar as theory of mind deficits would make it the case that they *could not* be deceitful in most cases, this would violate the principle that *ought implies can*. Thus, Kant would hardly praise autistic truthfulness. Of course, some persons with autism might attempt to be deceitful, but simply be very bad at it, owing to theory of mind deficits. If this is the case, then this again raises the question of the applicability of Kantian moral theory to the autistic agent.

8. See also Stanghellini 2001, especially pages 296–297, in which he adopts a Hegelian conception that without the ability to perform actions *qua* agent, the self loses the ability to come to know itself.

9. Goldman (2006) even questions the implementation of rationalist theories such as the first formulation of the categorical imperative for persons with ST deficits. Goldman claims that the third-person perspective required to, for example, act only on that maxim that thou canst at the same time will to be a universal law of nature—as well as that required for other moral theories, such as a Golden Rule, or to utilize thought experiments, such as the Original Position—are not available to those who cannot use ST.

10. Gene Pendleton (personal communication) asks whether this "should" is a moral "should," or whether it is of some other type. Two alternatives present themselves: (1) this is a prudential "should," or (2) this is an aesthetic "should." If it is a prudential "should," this raises the question "For whose sake is the cure being administered?" It may be for the sake

of the family and friends of the autistic person, but what of the autistic person himself? If he is otherwise happy, such that his prudential interests are satisfied, it is not clear that the prudential interests of the non-autistic persons should outweigh his prudential interests. Whose interests *should* prevail—the interests of the autistic person or the non-autistic persons? This question comes back to a moral question, and thus the initial "should" appears, at bottom, to be a moral question after all. Perhaps the initial "should" is somewhat like an aesthetic "should": the integrity of what a human being is is compromised when a human being does not have, in Nussbaum's terminology, all of the functional capabilities that make someone human. Thus, the autistic person should be cured, not out of a moral obligation, but out of a sense that this is what must be done to make him "whole." Analogies can be conjured up in which an autistic person who is cured is like a table whose last leg is attached before it is complete. The problem with this position is that in trying to restore a set of basic human capacities, the very humanness of the person who is being "restored" is not sufficiently taken into account. People are not tables. Barring another possibility, "Should an autistic adult be cured?" is a moral question after all.

4. Autism and Genetic Technologies

1. One question not addressed here is the question of genetic privacy, given that the primary evidence for a genetic basis for autism is based on studies of family history.

2. There is a sad irony in accepting the position that autism is more "socially acceptable" than mental retardation. It would appear that it is more socially acceptable when people are cut off from social relationships, as long as they are not cut off from objects, certain types of intellectual, or academic endeavors. Perhaps the "acceptable" nature of autism stems from a widespread ignorance about the ways in which autism does compromise an individual's relationships with others. However, if it is not the case that people are ignorant about the distinction between autism and mental retardation, a sad consequence emerges. The fact that it may be more palatable that a son or daughter is unable to have fulfilling reciprocal relationships, and less palatable that the same child has mental retardation, is a depressing statement about parental priorities.

3. Allen Buchanan et al. discuss such justifications (Buchanan et al. 2000, 54), but do not themselves endorse these justifications.

4. A question related to the questions discussed in this chapter about parents' choices to have children who are autistic is one raised by Jim Robinson (personal communication): would it be morally permissible to sterilize persons with autism who are unable to raise children, but who nonetheless are physically capable of having children? Given some of the arguments later in the chapter, it could be argued that it would be a violation of a child's right to an open future to be raised by autistic parents, or even one autistic parent. However, other ethical principles would supersede this concern: widespread sterilization of autistic persons would be a morally grotesque violation of justice, akin to the forced sterilizations practiced throughout the United States under eugenic policies. See note 6, below.

5. Whether Nussbaum is correct that persons with autism, including those with Asperger's syndrome, *can* attain the capabilities that she has evaluated as humanly central is discussed in chapter 2.

6. One of the interesting implications of the fact that the right to an open future argument may not be persuasive to autistic persons is that this argument may not have any bearing on the autistic person who chooses to have a child.

7. Davis (2001) observes that for these reasons Fletcher and Wertz (1990) have argued against telling parents the sex of their fetus.

5. Research on Persons with Autism

1. Beals's (2003) critique of this practice is singularly apt. See also McGovern (2006).

2. According to section 46.102(i) of the Common Rule, "minimal risk" means that "the probability and magnitude of harm or discomfort anticipated in the research are not greater in and of themselves than those ordinarily encountered in daily life or during the performance of routine physical or psychological examinations or tests" (Department of Health and Human Services 2005).

3. Waivers of informed consent are morally controversial, but some research cannot be accomplished if informed consent is offered prior to the research. One example is behavioral research that employs deception, in which the very fact that a behavior is being observed may affect the participant's behaviors, such that full informed consent will undermine the validity of the experiment. A second example is emergency research during a narrow therapeutic window in which the condition that qualifies a subject as a potential participant, such as stroke or head trauma, cannot be known before the event and affects decision making capacity. The ethical complexities of experiments that waive informed consent are not unique to persons with autism.

4. Buchanan and Brock explicitly state that their discussion is limited to decision making for medical treatment, and not for medical research (Buchanan and Brock 1990, 2). However, while they do observe some distinctions in the ethical landscape between treatment and research—the greater likelihood that the interests of researchers will deviate from the interests of subjects than will the interests of healthcare providers deviate from the interests of their patients (Buchanan and Brock 1990, 76) is one example—their observations about consent and capacities hold for both treatment and research.

5. There are a few exceptions to this claim, notable for their extraordinary circumstances. For example, participants in a biomedical experiment may not experience any risks by virtue of being in the experiment, but their future children may. Another exception includes some sorts of genetic research, in which the results of a genetic test may result in risks not merely to the subject who has undergone the study, but may place the family members or other members of the community who share a particular genetic trait at risk of loss of insurability by virtue of the knowledge that is gained from the study. A third exception could include xenotransplantation studies, in which previously unknown pathogens cross from one species into humans, from research subjects (who first bear the risks) to other non-subjects. Other elaborate examples could be contrived. The point in constructing such elaborate examples, however, is that these are the exceptions that prove the rule: research risks are borne primarily by the subjects themselves, whereas the benefits of research may or may not accrue to the subjects.

6. In a logical extension of the claim that therapeutic research is believed to be less controversial than non-therapeutic research, David Orentlicher argues that research should in some cases be a requirement of treatment: "linking treatment to participation in research could be a valuable and ethically sound way to increase patient participation, as long as the clinical trial involves a comparison of alternative, established therapies" (Orentlicher 2005, 21).

7. Asperger's syndrome is not charmingly "little professor syndrome" (Osborne 2000); "enchantment" does not appropriately describe autism any more than any other disability (Frith 2003).

Bibliography

Adshead, Gwen. 1999. Psychopaths and Other-Regarding Beliefs. *Philosophy, Psychiatry, & Psychology* 6(1): 41–44.

Ainslie, Donald C. 2002. Bioethics and the Problem of Pluralism. In *Bioethics*, ed. Ellen Frankel Paul, Fred D. Miller Jr., and Jeffrey Paul, 1–28. New York: Cambridge University Press.

American Academy of Pediatrics Committee of Children with Disabilities. 1998. Auditory Integration Training and Facilitated Communication for Autism. *Pediatrics* 102(2): 431–433.

American Psychiatric Association. 1994. *Diagnostic and Statistical Manual of Mental Disorders*, 4th ed. Washington, D.C.: American Psychiatric Association.

Andrews, Kristin. 2002. Interpreting Autism: A Critique of Davidson on Thought and Language. *Philosophical Psychology* 15(3): 317–332.

Andrews, Kristin, and Ljiljana Radenovic. 2006. Speaking without Interpreting: A Reply to Bouma on Autism and Davidsonian Interpretation. *Philosophical Psychology* 19(5): 663–678.

Appelbaum, Paul S., Loren H. Roth, Charles W. Lidz, et al. 1987. False Hopes and Best Data: Consent to Research and the Therapeutic Misconception. *Hastings Center Report* 17(2): 20–24.

Aristotle. 1955. *The Ethics of Aristotle: The Nicomachean Ethics.* Trans. J. A. K. Thomson. Middlesex: Penguin Books.

Asch, Adrienne. 1995. Genetics and Employment: More Disability Discrimination. In *The Human Genome Project and the Future of Health Care*, ed. Thomas H. Murray, Mark A. Rothstein, and Robert F. Murray Jr., 158–172. Bloomington: Indiana University Press.

———. 2000. Why I Haven't Changed My Mind about Prenatal Diagnosis: Reflections and Refinements. In *Prenatal Testing and Disability Rights*, ed. Erik Parens and Adrienne Asch, 234–258. Washington, D.C.: Georgetown University Press.

———. 2003. Prenatal Diagnosis and Selective Abortion: A Challenge to Practice and Policy. In *Ethical Issues in Modern Medicine*, 6th ed., ed. Bonnie Steinbock, John D. Arras, and Alex John London, 523–533. New York: McGraw-Hill.

Aune, Bruce. 1979. *Kant's Theory of Morals.* Princeton, N.J.: Princeton University Press.

Autism Genome Project Consortium. 2007. Mapping Autism Risk Loci Using Genetic Linkage and Chromosomal Rearrangements. *Nature Genetics* 39(3): 319–328, corrigendum 39(10): 1285.

Barker, John A. 1997. Review of Mindblindness: An Essay on Autism and Theory of Mind, by Simon Baron-Cohen. *Philosophical Psychology* 10(2): 256–257.

———. 2002. Computer Modeling and the Fate of Folk Psychology. *Metaphilosophy* 33(1&2): 30–48.

Barnbaum, Deborah R. 2001. Response to Gina Kolata's "Fertility Expert Approves Couples Choosing the Sex of Their Embryos." *BIO Quarterly* 11(4): 3.

Barnbaum, Deborah R., and Michael Byron, eds. 2001. *Research Ethics: Text and Readings*. Upper Saddle River, N.J.: Prentice Hall.

Baron-Cohen, Simon. 1995. *Mindblindness: An Essay on Autism and Theory of Mind*. Cambridge, Mass.: MIT Press.

———. 1999. Can Studies of Autism Teach Us about Consciousness of the Physical and the Mental? *Philosophical Explorations* 2(3): 175–188.

———. 2000a. Autism: Deficits in Folk Psychology Exist Alongside Superiority in Folk Physics. In *Understanding Other Minds: Perspectives from Developmental Cognitive Neuroscience*, 2nd ed., ed. Simon Baron-Cohen, Helen Tager-Flusberg, and Donald J. Cohen, 74–82. New York: Oxford University Press.

———. 2000b. Theory of Mind and Autism: A Fifteen Year Review. In *Understanding Other Minds: Perspectives from Developmental Cognitive Neuroscience*, 2nd ed., ed. Simon Baron-Cohen, Helen Tager-Flusberg, and Donald J. Cohen, 3–20. New York: Oxford University Press.

———. 2003. *The Essential Difference: The Truth about the Male & Female Brain*. New York: Basic Books.

Baron-Cohen, Simon, and Patrick Bolton. 1993. *Autism: The Facts*. New York: Oxford University Press.

Bazelon, Emily. 2007. What Autistic Girls Are Made Of. *New York Times Magazine*, August 5.

Beals, Katharine P. 2003. The Ethics of Autism: What's Wrong with the Dominant Paradigms and How to Fix Them. *Mental Retardation and Developmental Disabilities Research Reviews* 9: 32–39.

Beauchamp, Tom L., and James F. Childress. 2001. *Principles of Biomedical Ethics*, 5th ed. New York: Oxford University Press.

Benn, Piers. 1999. Freedom, Resentment, and the Psychopath. *Philosophy, Psychiatry, & Psychology* 6(1): 29–39.

Bernier, Paul. 2002. From Simulation to Theory. In *Simulation and Knowledge of Action*, ed. Jérôme Dokic and Joëlle Proust, 33–48. Philadelphia: John Benjamins.

Billstedt, Eva, Carina Gillberg, and Christopher Gillberg. 2005. Autism after Adolescence: Population-Based 13-to 22-Year Follow-Up Study of 120 Individuals with Autism Diagnosed in Childhood. *Journal of Autism and Developmental Disorders* 35(3): 351–360.

Blair, R. James R. 1996. Brief Report: Morality in the Autistic Child. *Journal of Autism and Developmental Disorders* 26(5): 571–579.

Blum, Lawrence A. 1991. Moral Perception and Particularity. *Ethics* 101(4): 701–725.

Botz-Bornstein, Thorsten. 2004. Virtual Reality and Dreams: Towards the Autistic Condition? *Philosophy in the Contemporary World* 11(2): 1–10.

Bouma, Hanni K. 2006a. High-Functioning Autistic Speakers as Davidsonian Interpreters: A Reply to Andrews and Radenovic. *Philosophical Psychology* 19(5): 679–690.

———. 2006b. Radical Interpretation and High-Functioning Autistic Speakers: A Defense of Davidson on Thought and Language. *Philosophical Psychology* 19(5): 639–662.

Brentano, Franz C. 1973. *Psychology from an Empirical Standpoint.* Ed. Oskar Kraus, trans. Antos Rancurello, Dailey Burnham Terrell, and Linda L. McAlister. New York: Humanities Press.

Brandt, Richard B. 1992. *Morality, Utilitarianism, and Rights.* New York: Cambridge University Press.

Brown, Barry F. 2006. Proxy Consent for Research on the Incompetent Elderly. In *Biomedical Ethics,* 6th ed., ed. Thomas A. Mappes and David DeGrazia, 240–247. New York: McGraw-Hill.

Buber, Martin. 2002. *The Martin Buber Reader: Essential Writings.* Ed. Asher D. Biemann. New York: Palgrave Macmillan.

Buchanan, Allen E. 1996. Choosing Who Will Be Disabled: Genetic Intervention and the Morality of Inclusion. *Social Philosophy and Policy* 13: 18–46.

Buchanan, Allen E., and Dan W. Brock. 1990. *Deciding for Others: The Ethics of Surrogate Decision Making.* New York: Cambridge University Press.

Buchanan, Allen E., Dan W. Brock, Norman Daniels, and Daniel Wikler. 2000. *From Chance to Choice: Genetics & Justice.* New York: Cambridge University Press.

Campbell, Daniel B., James S. Sutcliffe, Philip J. Ebert, et al. 2006. A Genetic Variant That Disrupts *MET* Transcription Is Associated with Autism. *Proceedings of the National Academy of Sciences* 103(45): 16834–16839.

Caplan, Arthur L. 1997. The Concepts of Health, Illness, and Disease. In *Medical Ethics,* ed. Robert M. Veatch, 57–74. Sudbury: Jones and Bartlett.

Carey, Benedict. 2004. To Treat Autism, Parents Take a Leap of Faith. *New York Times,* December 27, Health Desk.

———. 2007. Study Puts Rates of Autism at 1 in 150 U.S. Children. *New York Times,* February 9, correction Feb. 10, 2007, Health Desk.

Charman, Tony. 2000. Theory of Mind and the Early Diagnosis of Autism. In *Understanding Other Minds: Perspectives from Developmental Cognitive Neuroscience,* 2nd ed., ed. Simon Baron-Cohen, Helen Tager-Flusberg, and Donald J. Cohen, 423–441. New York: Oxford University Press.

Chen, Donna T., Franklin G. Miller, and Donald L. Rosenstein. 2003. Ethical Aspects of Research Into the Etiology of Autism. *Mental Retardation and Developmental Disabilities Research Reviews* 9: 48–53.

Coltheart, Max. 1999. Modularity and Cognition. *Trends in Cognitive Sciences* 3(3): 115–120.

Coltheart, Max, and Robyn Langdon. 1998. Autism, Modularity and Levels of Explanation in Cognitive Science. *Mind & Language* 13(1): 138–152.

Cone, Marla. 2007. PCBs Cause Autism-Like Condition in Newborn Rats. *Los Angeles Times,* April 25, National Desk.

Croen, Lisa A., Judith K. Grether, Jenny Hoogstrate, and Steve Selvin. 2002. The Changing Prevalence of Autism in California. *Journal of Autism and Developmental Disorders* 32(3): 207–215.

Daly, Emma. 2005. Manhattan Charter School to Serve the Autistic. *New York Times*, May 4, New York/Region Desk.

Dancy, Jonathan. 1993. *Moral Reasons*. Oxford: Blackwell.

———. 2000. The Particularist's Progress. In *Moral Particularism*, ed. Brad Hooker and Margaret Olivia Little, 130–156. New York: Oxford University Press.

Davidson, Donald. 1984a. Belief and the Basis of Meaning. In *Inquiries into Truth and Interpretation*, 141–154. Oxford: Clarendon.

———. 1984b. Radical Interpretation. In *Inquiries into Truth and Interpretation*, 125–140. Oxford: Clarendon.

———. 2005. The Social Aspect of Language. In *Truth, Language, and History*, 109–126. New York: Oxford University Press.

Davis, Dena S. 2001. *Genetic Dilemmas: Reproductive Technology, Parental Choices, and Children's Futures*. New York: Routledge.

Dennett, Daniel C. 1987. *The Intentional Stance*. Cambridge, Mass.: MIT Press.

Department of Health and Human Services, National Institutes of Health, and Office for Human Research Protections. 2005. The Common Rule, Title 45 (Public Welfare), Code of Federal Regulations, Part 46 (Protection of Human Subjects), http://www.hhs.gov/ohrp/humansubjects/guidance/45cfr46.htm (accessed January 4, 2008).

de Villiers, Jill. 2000. Language and Theory of Mind: What Are the Developmental Relationships? In *Understanding Other Minds: Perspectives from Developmental Cognitive Neuroscience*, 2nd ed., ed. Simon Baron-Cohen, Helen Tager-Flusberg, and Donald J. Cohen, 84–123. New York: Oxford University Press.

Dworkin, Gerald. 1988. *The Theory and Practice of Autonomy*. New York: Cambridge University Press.

Erevelles, Nirmala. 2002. Voices of Silence: Foucault, Disability, and the Question of Self-Determination. *Studies in Philosophy and Education* 21(1): 17–35.

Evnine, Simon. 1991. *Donald Davidson*. Stanford: Stanford University Press.

Feinberg, Joel. 1980. The Child's Right to an Open Future. In *Whose Child? Children's Rights, Parental Authority, and State Power*, ed. William Aiken and Hugh LaFollette, 124–153. Totowa, N.J.: Rowman and Littlefield.

Fisher, Celia B. 2003. Goodness-of-Fit Ethic for Informed Consent to Research Involving Adults with Mental Retardation and Developmental Disabilities. *Mental Retardation and Developmental Disabilities Research Reviews* 9: 27–31.

Fletcher, John C., and Dorothy C. Wertz. 1990. Ethics, Law, and Medical Genetics. *Emory Law Journal* 39: 747–809.

Fletcher, Joseph. 1972. Indicators of Humanhood: A Tentative Profile of Man. *Hastings Center Report* 2(5): 1–4.

Fodor, Jerry A. 1983. *The Modularity of Mind*. Cambridge, Mass.: MIT Press.

Freudenheim, Milt. 2004. Battling Insurers Over Autism Treatment. *New York Times*, December 21, Business Desk.

Frey, R. G., ed. 1984. *Utility and Rights*. Minneapolis: University of Minnesota Press.

Frith, Uta. 2003. *Autism: Explaining the Enigma*, 2nd ed. Oxford: Blackwell.

Frith, Uta, and Francesca Happé. 1999. Theory of Mind and Self-Consciousness: What Is It Like to Be Autistic? *Mind & Language* 14(1): 1–22.

Gallagher, Shaun. 2004. Understanding Interpersonal Problems in Autism: Interaction Theory as an Alternative to Theory of Mind. *Philosophy, Psychiatry, & Psychology* 11(3): 199–217.

Garfield, Jay L. 2000. Particularity and Principle: The Structure of Moral Knowledge. In *Moral Particularism*, ed. Brad Hooker and Margaret Olivia Little, 178–204. New York: Oxford University Press.

Garfield, Jay L., Candida C. Peterson, and Tricia Perry. 2001. Social Cognition, Language Acquisition and the Development of the Theory of Mind. *Mind & Language* 16(5): 494–541.

Gerland, Gunilla. 1996. *A Real Person: Life on the Outside*. Trans. Joan Tate. London: Souvenir Press.

Gerrans, Philip. 2002. The Theory of Mind Module in Evolutionary Psychology. *Biology and Philosophy* 17(3): 305–321.

Gert, Bernard, Charles M. Culver, and K. Danner Clouser. 1997. *Bioethics: A Return to Fundamentals*. New York: Oxford University Press.

Ghaziuddin, Mohammad. 2005. A Family History Study of Asperger Syndrome. *Journal of Autism and Developmental Disorders* 35(2): 177–182.

Gibbs, Paul J. 1988. Autism in Low-Functioning Subjects: Early Environment and the Theory of Mind Deficit. *Contemporary Philosophy* 20(5–6): 3–9.

Gipps, Richard. 2004. Autism and Intersubjectivity: Beyond Cognitivism and the Theory of Mind. *Philosophy, Psychiatry, & Psychology* 11(3): 195–198.

Glüer, Kathrin, and Peter Pagin. 2003. Meaning Theory and Autistic Speakers. *Mind & Language* 18(1): 23–51.

Goldman, Alvin I. 2002. Simulation Theory and Mental Concepts. In *Simulation and Knowledge of Action*, ed. Jérôme Dokic and Joëlle Proust, 1–20. Philadelphia: John Benjamins.

———. 2006. *Simulating Minds: The Philosophy, Psychology, and Neuroscience of Mindreading*. New York: Oxford University Press.

Goode, Erica. 2004a. Autism Cases Up; Cause Is Unclear. *New York Times,* January 26, U.S. Desk.

———. 2004b. Lifting the Veils of Autism, One by One by One. *New York Times,* February 24, Science Desk.

Gopnik, Alison, Lisa Capps, and Andrew Meltzoff. 2000. Early Theories of Mind: What the Theory Theory Can Tell Us about Autism. In *Understanding Other Minds: Perspectives from Developmental Cognitive Neuroscience*, 2nd ed., ed. Simon Baron-Cohen, Helen Tager-Flusberg, and Donald J. Cohen, 50–72. New York: Oxford University Press.

Gordon, Robert M., and John A. Barker. 1994. Autism and the "Theory of Mind" Debate. In *Philosophical Psychopathology*, ed. George Graham and G. Lynn Stephens, 163–181. Cambridge, Mass.: MIT Press.

Graham, George, and G. Lynn Stephens, eds. 1994. *Philosophical Psychopathology*. Cambridge, Mass.: MIT Press.

Graham, Gordon. 2001. Music and Autism. *Journal of Aesthetic Education* 35(2): 39–47.

Grandin, Temple. 1995. *Thinking in Pictures and Other Reports from My Life with Autism.* New York: Doubleday.

Grant, Cathy M., Jill Boucher, Kevin J. Riggs, and Andrew Grayson. 2005. Moral Understanding in Children with Autism. *Autism* 9(3): 317–331.

Green, Ronald M. 1997. Parental Autonomy and the Obligation Not to Harm One's Child Genetically. *Journal of Law, Medicine, and Ethics* 25(1): 5–15.

Grice, H. P. 1957. Meaning. *The Philosophical Review* 66(3): 377–388.

Gross, Jane. 2005. As Autistic Children Grow, So Does Social Gap. *New York Times,* February 26, Health Desk.

Guttenplan, Samuel. Modularity. In *A Companion to the Philosophy of Mind,* ed. Samuel Guttenplan, 441–449. Oxford: Blackwell.

Happé, Francesca. 2000. Parts and Wholes, Meaning and Minds: Central Coherence and Its Relation to Theory of Mind. In *Understanding Other Minds: Perspectives from Developmental Cognitive Neuroscience,* 2nd ed., ed. Simon Baron-Cohen, Helen Tager-Flusberg, and Donald J. Cohen, 203–221. New York: Oxford University Press.

Happé, Francesca, and Uta Frith. 2006. The Weak Central Coherence Account: Detail-Focused Cognitive Style in Autism Spectrum Disorders. *Journal of Autism and Developmental Disorders* 36(1): 5–25.

Harmon, Amy. 2004. How about Not "Curing" Us, Some Autistics Are Pleading. *New York Times,* December 20, Health Desk.

Harris, Gardiner. 2005. No Vaccine-Autism Link, Parents Are Told. *New York Times,* July 20, Health Desk.

Harris, Gardiner, and Anahad O'Connor. 2005. On Autism's Cause, It's Parents vs. Research. *New York Times,* June 25, Health Desk.

Hellman, Samuel, and Deborah S. Hellman. 2001. Of Mice but Not Men: Problems of the Randomized Clinical Trial. In *Research Ethics: Text and Readings,* ed. Deborah R. Barnbaum and Michael Byron, 58–64. Upper Saddle River, N.J.: Prentice Hall.

Herba, Catherine M., Sheilagh Hodgins, Nigel Blackwood, et al. 2007. The Neurobiology of Psychopathy: A Focus on Emotion Processing. In *The Psychopath: Theory, Research, and Practice,* ed. Hugues Hervé and John C. Yuille, 253–286. Mahwah, N.J.: Lawrence Erlbaum.

Hervé, Hugues. 2007. Psychopathy Across the Ages: A History of the Hare Psychopath. In *The Psychopath: Theory, Research, and Practice,* ed. Hugues Hervé and John C. Yuille, 31–56. Mahwah, N.J.: Lawrence Erlbaum.

Hick, John. 1977. *Evil and the God of Love.* San Francisco: Harper and Row.

Hobson, R. Peter. 1993. The Emotional Origins of Social Understanding. *Philosophical Psychology* 6(3): 227–249.

Hooker, Brad, and Margaret Olivia Little, eds. 2000. *Moral Particularism.* New York: Oxford University Press.

Howlin, Patricia, Susan Goode, Jane Hutton, and Michael Rutter. 2004. Adult Outcomes for Children with Autism. *Journal of Child Psychology and Psychiatry* 45(2): 212–229.

Hume, David. 1948. A Treatise of Human Nature and An Enquiry Concerning Human Understanding. In Moral and Political Philosophy. Ed. Henry D. Aiken. New York: MacMillan.

Hutto, David D. 2003. Folk Psychological Narratives and the Case of Autism. *Philosophical Papers* 32(3): 315–361.

Kamawar, Deepthi, Jay L. Garfield, and Jill de Villiers. 2002. Coherence as an Explanation for Theory of Mind Task Failure in Autism. *Mind & Language* 17(3): 266–272.

Kanner, Leo. 1943. Autistic Disturbances of Affective Contact. *Nervous Child* 2: 217–250.

Kant, Immanuel. 1956. *Groundwork of the Metaphysic of Morals*. Trans. H. J. Paton. New York: Harper and Row.

Kennett, Jeanette. 2002. Autism, Empathy and Moral Agency. *The Philosophical Quarterly* 52(208): 340–357.

Khamsi, Roxanne. 2006. Emotion Centre of Autistic Brains Have Fewer Cells. *Newscientist.com*, July 19, http://www.newscientist.com/article/dn9578.html (accessed January 4, 2008).

King, Nancy M. P. 2000. Defining and Describing Benefit Appropriately in Clinical Trials. *Journal of Law, Medicine, and Ethics* 28(4): 332–343.

Kittay, Eva Feder. 2005. At the Margins of Moral Personhood. *Ethics* 116(1): 100–131.

Kotsopoulos, Sotiris. 2000. Uncertainties in Aetiology and Treatment of Infantile Autism—Assumptions and Evidence. *Medicine, Health Care, and Philosophy* 3(2): 175–178.

Kuehn, Bridget M. 2006. Studies Probe Autism Anatomy, Genetics. *Journal of the American Medical Association* 295(1): 19–20.

Langdon, Robyn. 2003. Theory of Mind and Social Dysfunction: Psychotic Solipsism Versus Autistic Asociality. In *Individual Differences in Theory of Mind: Implications for Typical and Atypical Development*, ed. Betty Repacholi and Virginia Slaughter, 241–269. New York: Psychology Press.

Lawson, John. 2003. Depth Accessibility Difficulties: An Alternative Conceptualisation of Autism Spectrum Conditions. *Journal for the Theory of Social Behaviour* 33(2): 189–202.

Lawson, Wendy. 1998. *Life Behind Glass: A Personal Account of Autism Spectrum Disorder*. Philadelphia: Jessica Kingsley.

Lewis, David. 1969. *Convention: A Philosophical Study*. Oxford: Blackwell.

Livet, Pierre. 2002. Reply to Donald M. Peterson. In *Simulation and Knowledge of Action*, ed. Jérôme Dokic and Joëlle Proust, 197–200. Philadelphia: John Benjamins.

McGeer, Victoria. 2001. Psycho-Practice, Psycho-Theory and the Contrastive Case of Autism: How Practices of Mind Become Second-Nature. *Journal of Consciousness Studies* 8(5–7): 109–132.

———. 2004. Autistic Self-Awareness. *Philosophy, Psychiatry, & Psychology* 11(3): 235–251.

———. 2005. Out of the Mouths of Autistics. In *Cognition and the Brain: The Philosophy and Neuroscience Movement*, ed. Andrew Brook and Kathleen Akins, 98–127. New York: Cambridge University Press.

McGovern, Cammie. 2006. Autism's Parent Trap. *New York Times*, June 5, Opinion Desk.

McMahan, Jeff. 2005. Causing Disabled People to Exist and Causing People to Be Disabled. *Ethics* 116(1): 77–99.

Mill, John Stuart. 1979. *Utilitarianism*. Ed. George Sher. Indianapolis: Hackett.

Minkowski, Eugène, and R. Targowla. 2001. A Contribution to the Study of Autism: The Interrogative Attitude. *Philosophy, Psychiatry, & Psychology* 8(4): 271–278.

Monastersky, Richard. 2007. Genetics Researchers Tie Autism to Specific Parts of Chromosomes. *The Chronicle of Higher Education,* February 20, http://chronicle.com/daily/2007/02/2007022003n.htm (accessed January 4, 2008; subscription required).

Moore, Abigail Sullivan. 2006. A Dream Not Denied: Students on the Spectrum. *New York Times,* November 5, Education Life Desk.

Murray, Thomas H. 1996. *The Worth of a Child.* Berkeley and Los Angeles: University of California Press.

National Commission for the Protection of Human Subjects of Biomedical and Behavioral Research. 1978. *The Belmont Report.* Washington, D.C.: Department of Health, Education, and Welfare.

Nelson, James Lindemann. 2000. The Meaning of the Act: Reflections on the Expressive Force of Reproductive Decision Making and Policies. In *Prenatal Testing and Disability Rights,* ed. Erik Parens and Adrienne Asch, 196–213. Washington, D.C.: Georgetown University Press.

Nichols, Shaun. 2004. *Sentimental Rules: On the Natural Foundation of Moral Judgment.* New York: Oxford University Press.

Nichols, Shaun, and Stephen Stich. 1998. Rethinking Co-Cognition: A Reply to Heal. *Mind & Language* 13(4): 499–512.

———. 2003. How to Read Your Own Mind: A Cognitive Theory of Self-Consciousness. In *Consciousness: New Philosophical Perspectives,* ed. Quentin Smith and Aleksandar Jokic, 157–200. New York: Oxford University Press.

Noonan, John. 1968. Deciding Who Is Human. *Natural Law Forum* 13: 134–138.

Nussbaum, Martha C. 1995. Human Capabilities, Female Human Beings. In *Women, Culture and Development,* ed. Martha C. Nussbaum and Jonathan Glover, 61–104. New York: Oxford University Press.

———. 2006. *Frontiers of Justice: Disability, Nationality, Species Membership.* Cambridge, Mass.: The Belknap Press of Harvard University Press.

O'Loughlin, Claire, and Paul Thagard. 2000. Autism and Coherence: A Conceptual Model. *Mind & Language* 15(4): 375–392.

O'Neill, Onora. 2002. *Autonomy and Trust in Bioethics.* New York: Cambridge University Press.

Orentlicher, David. 2005. Making Research a Requirement of Treatment: Why We Should Sometimes Let Doctors Pressure Patients to Participate in Research. *Hastings Center Report* 35(5): 20–28.

Osborne, Lawrence. 2000. The Little Professor Syndrome. *New York Times Magazine,* June 18.

Parens, Erik, and Adrienne Asch, eds. 2000. *Prenatal Testing and Disability Rights.* Washington, D.C.: Georgetown University Press.

Parfit, Derek. 1984. *Reasons and Persons.* Oxford: Clarendon.

Parnas, Josef. 2004. Belief and Pathology of Self-Awareness: A Phenomenological Contribution to the Classification of Delusions. *Journal of Consciousness Studies* 11(10–11): 148–161.

Perner, Josef, and Birgit Lang. 2000. Theory of Mind and Executive Function: Is There a Developmental Relationship? In *Understanding Other Minds: Perspectives from Developmental Cognitive Neuroscience,* 2nd ed., ed. Simon Baron-Cohen, Helen Tager-Flusberg, and Donald J. Cohen, 150–181. New York: Oxford University Press.

Peterson, Donald M. 2002. Mental Simulation, Dialogical Processing and the Syndrome of Autism. In *Simulation and Knowledge of Action,* ed. Jérôme Dokic and Joëlle Proust, 185–195. Philadelphia: John Benjamins.

Phillips, Wendy, Simon Baron-Cohen, and Michael Rutter. 1998. Understanding Intention in Normal Development and in Autism. *British Journal of Developmental Psychology* 16: 337–348.

Plaisted, Kate. 2000. Aspects of Autism that Theory of Mind Cannot Easily Explain. In *Understanding Other Minds: Perspectives from Developmental Cognitive Neuroscience,* 2nd ed., ed. Simon Baron-Cohen, Helen Tager-Flusberg, and Donald J. Cohen, 223–249. New York: Oxford University Press.

Plato. 1974. *Republic.* Trans. G. M. A. Grube. Indianapolis: Hackett.

Ponnet, Koen, Ann Buysse, Herbert Roeyers, and Kim De Corte. 2005. Empathic Accuracy in Adults with a Pervasive Developmental Disorder During an Unstructured Conversation with a Typically Developing Stranger. *Journal of Autism and Developmental Disorders* 35(5): 585–600.

Purdy, Laura M. 2006. Genetics and Reproductive Risk: Can Having Children Be Immoral? In *Biomedical Ethics,* 6th ed., ed. Thomas A. Mappes and David DeGrazia, 526–532. Boston: McGraw-Hill.

Raffman, Diana. 1999. What Autism May Tell Us about Self-Consciousness: A Commentary on Frith and Happé. *Mind & Language* 14(1): 23–31.

Ramachandran, Vilayanur S., and Lindsay M. Oberman. 2006. Broken Mirrors: A Theory of Autism. *Scientific American,* November.

Ramberg, Bjørn T. 1989. *Donald Davidson's Philosophy of Language: An Introduction.* Oxford: Blackwell.

Reuters News Service. 2007. Debate Over Vaccines' Role in Autism Heads to a Court. *Wall Street Journal,* June 11: B7.

Ross, David. 2002. *The Right and the Good.* Ed. Phillip Stratton-Lake. New York: Oxford University Press.

Ruddick, William. 2000. Ways to Limit Prenatal Testing. In *Prenatal Testing and Disability Rights,* ed. Erik Parens and Adrienne Asch, 95–107. Washington, D.C.: Georgetown University Press.

Sacks, Oliver. 1995. *An Anthropologist on Mars.* New York: Vintage.

Scanlon, Thomas M.. 1998. *What We Owe to Each Other.* Cambridge, Mass.: The Belknap Press of Harvard University Press.

Scheurich, Neil. 2002. Moral Attitudes and Mental Disorders. *Hastings Center Report* 32(2): 14–21.

Scholl, Brian J., and Alan M. Leslie. 1999. Modularity, Development, and "Theory of Mind." *Mind & Language* 14(1): 131–153.

Schumann, Cynthia Mills, and David G. Amaral. 2006. Stereological Analysis of Amygdala Neuron Number in Autism. *The Journal of Neuroscience* 26(29): 7674–7679.

Sen, Amartya. 1991. Rights and Agency. In *Consequentialism and Its Critics,* ed. Samuel Scheffler, 187–223. New York: Oxford University Press.

Shanker, Stuart. 2004. Autism and the Dynamic Developmental Model of Emotions. *Philosophy, Psychiatry, & Psychology* 11(3): 219–233.

Shattuck, Paul T. 2006. The Contribution of Diagnostic Substitution to the Growing Administrative Prevalence of Autism in US Special Education. *Pediatrics* 117(4): 1028–1037.

Shoemaker, David. 2007. Moral Address, Moral Responsibility, and the Boundaries of the Moral Community. *Ethics* 118(1): 70–108.

Siegel, Bryna. 1996. *The World of the Autistic Child: Understanding and Treating Autistic Spectrum Disorders.* New York: Oxford University Press.

Sinclair, Jim. 1992. Bridging the Gaps: An Inside-Out View of Autism (Or, Do You Know What I Don't Know?). In *High-Functioning Individuals with Autism,* ed. Eric Schopler and Gary B. Mesibov, 294–302. New York: Plenum Press.

Smetana, Judith G. 1985. Preschool Children's Conceptions of Transgressions: Effects of Varying Moral and Conventional Domain-Related Attributes. *Developmental Psychology* 21(1): 18–29.

Snyder, Allan W. 1998. Breaking Mindset. *Mind & Language* 13(1): 1–10.

Stanghellini, Giovanni. 2001. A Dialectical Conception of Autism. *Philosophy, Psychiatry, & Psychology* 8(4): 295–298.

Steinbock, Bonnie. 2000. Disability, Prenatal Testing, and Selective Abortion. In *Prenatal Testing and Disability Rights,* ed. Erik Parens and Adrienne Asch, 108–124. Washington, D.C.: Georgetown University Press.

———. 2002. Sex Selection: Not Obviously Wrong. *Hastings Center Report* 32(1): 23–28.

Stich, Stephen, and Shaun Nichols. 1997. Cognitive Penetrability, Rationality, and Restricted Simulation. *Mind & Language* 12(3&4): 297–326.

Strawson, Peter F. 1970. *Meaning and Truth: An Inaugural Lecture Delivered Before the University of Oxford on November 5, 1969.* Oxford: Clarendon.

———. 1974. Freedom and Resentment. In *Freedom and Resentment, and Other Essays,* 5–13. London: Methuen.

Stueber, Karsten R. 2006. *Rediscovering Empathy: Agency, Folk Psychology, and the Human Sciences.* Cambridge, Mass.: MIT Press.

Sullivan, Roger J. 1989. *Immanuel Kant's Moral Theory.* New York: Cambridge University Press.

Szatmari, Peter A. 2004. *A Mind Apart: Understanding Children with Autism and Asperger Syndrome.* New York: Guilford Press.

Tarksi, Alfred. 1956. The Concept of Truth in Formalized Languages. In *Logic, Semantics, Metamathematics: Papers from 1923 to 1938,* trans. J. H. Woodger, 152–278. Oxford: Clarendon.

Tager-Flusberg, Helen. 2003. Exploring the Relationship between Theory of Mind and Social-Communicative Functioning in Children with Autism. In *Individual Differences in Theory of Mind: Implications for Typical and Atypical Development,* ed. Betty Repacholi and Virginia Slaughter, 197–212. New York: Psychology Press.

Tager-Flusberg, Helen, and Robert M. Joseph. 2005. How Language Facilitates the Acquisition of False-Belief Understanding in Children with Autism. In *Why Language Matters for Theory of Mind*, ed. Janet Wilde Astington and Jodie A. Baird, 298–318. New York: Oxford University Press.

Thagard, Paul, and Claire O'Loughlin. 2002. False Photos, False Beliefs, and Coherence: A Response to Kamawar et al. *Mind & Language* 17(3): 273–275.

Veatch, Robert M. 1999. Abandoning Informed Consent. In *Bioethics: An Anthology*, ed. Helga Kuhse and Peter Singer, 523–532. Oxford: Blackwell.

Vitello, Paul. 2007. Being Nice to the Bacon, Before You Bring It Home. *New York Times*, April 1, Week in Review Desk.

Wade, Nicholas. 2007. Progress Is Reported on a Type of Autism. *New York Times*, February 20, Health Desk.

Warren, Mary Anne. 1996. On the Moral and Legal Status of Abortion. In *The Problem of Abortion*, 3rd ed., ed. Susan Dwyer and Joel Feinberg, 59–74. Belmont, Calif.: Wadsworth.

Wasserman, David. 2005. The Nonidentity Problem, Disability, and the Role Morality of Prospective Parents. *Ethics* 116(1): 132–152.

Williams, Donna. 1992. *Nobody Nowhere: The Extraordinary Autobiography of An Autistic*. New York: Avon.

———. 1994. *Somebody Somewhere: Breaking Free from the World of Autism*. New York: Times Books.

Williams, Justin H. G., Andrew Whiten, Thomas Suddendorf, and David I. Perrett. 2001. Imitation, Mirror Neurons and Autism. *Neuroscience and Biobehavioral Reviews* 25(4): 287–295.

Wimmer, Heinz, and Joseph Perner. 1983. Beliefs about Beliefs: Representation and Constraining Function of Wrong Beliefs in Young Children's Understanding of Deception. *Cognition* 13(1): 103–128.

Wolf, Susan. 1995. Commentary on Martha C. Nussbaum: Human Capabilities, Female Human Beings. In *Women, Culture and Development*, ed. Martha Nussbaum and Jonathan Glover, 105–115. New York: Oxford University Press.

World Health Organization. 1993. *International Statistical Classification of Diseases and Related Health Problems*, 10th revision. Geneva: World Health Organization.

World Medical Association. 2004. *Declaration of Helsinki: Ethical Principles for Medical Research Involving Human Subjects*. Tokyo: World Medical Association, http://www.wma.net/e/policy/b3.htm (accessed January 4, 2008).

Zilberberg, Julie M. 2004. A Boy or a Girl: Is Any Choice Moral? The Ethics of Sex Selection and Sex Preselection in Context. In *Linking Visions: Feminist Bioethics, Human Rights, and the Developing World*, ed. Rosemary Tong, Anne Donchin, and Susan Dodds, 147–156. Lanham, Md.: Rowman & Littlefield.

Index

Deborah R. Barnbaum is Associate Professor of Philosophy at Kent State University, specializing in bioethics, and Program Coordinator for Kent State University's and Northeastern Ohio Universities College of Medicine's combined BS/MD program. She is co-author of *Research Ethics: Text and Readings,* and publishes in journals such as *IRB: Ethics & Human Research, Politics and the Life Sciences,* and *The Journal of Applied Philosophy.* Barnbaum also engages hospitals with her scholarship, giving presentations, serving on ethics committees, and taking residents on rounds to discuss the ethical implications of cases.